HEALTH CARE MARKETING PLANS: FROM STRATEGY TO ACTION

HEALTH CARE MARKETING PLANS: FROM STRATEGY TO ACTION

Steven G. Hillestad
Eric N. Berkowitz

DOW JONES-IRWIN
Homewood, Illinois 60430

ISBN 0-87094-462-2

Library of Congress Catalog Card No. 83–71842

Printed in the United States of America

1 2 3 4 5 6 7 8 9 0 K 1 0 9 8 7 6 5 4

To Anne, Marcia, Sandra, Signe, and Theodore

"One senior executive made the important observation that getting the marketing concept understood and accepted is still the biggest challenge faced by any organization despite the fact that the concept is now more than a quarter of a century old.

"There was virtual unanimity among these executives that marketing is the critical management function in their firm from a strategic viewpoint, and it is likely to become more important in the current decade."

Frederick Webster, "Top Management's Concerns about Marketing Issues for the 1980s," *Journal of Marketing* 45 (Summer 1981), pp. 9–16.

FOREWORD

Many physicians and hospital presidents are seeking to take advantage of new business opportunities being created by constantly changing government regulations, the growing number of physicians, and more demanding consumers.

As a result of rapid changes in the supply and demand for health care services, America's health care providers are responding to consumers' demands for more recognition of their needs. They are developing and implementing product-line marketing strategies that answer the market's demand for convenient and low-cost services as well as for high-technology care.

Few hospitals, multihospital systems, nursing home chains, or physicians seriously considered the market's needs and wants before the late 1970s. Historically, they decided they wanted to offer their services and went into business without developing a marketing strategy. Although few hospitals or group practices went out of business, many languished. And too many of the services introduced without professional marketing plans are losing money today. They are losing money because their creators failed to evaluate pricing strategies and paid little attention to the strength of similar services offered by competitors. Under the cost-based reimbursement system, such mistakes could be hidden by subsidizing them with profits from profitable services.

But the era of cost-based reimbursements by Medicare and other insurers is history. Hospitals can no longer subsidize money-losing services with their winners. Under Medicare's prospective payment system, hospitals must deliver inpatient services for fixed prices. If a hospital's costs are less than the price Medicare has set for a diagnosis-related group of illnesses, it makes money on that DRG. When costs exceed Medicare's DRG price per case, a hospital loses money. It no longer pays to spend more to make more, unless an institution has a carefully prepared marketing strategy.

Health care providers are being forced to find their niches in the market. Being the low-cost producer is important. But it isn't enough. Like other businesses, hospitals and clinics must do their market research to learn what consumers want and need, and use the processes and questions in this book to develop and implement their marketing strategies.

In response to the business community's demand for lower-cost health care, some hospitals and clinics are packaging their services to cut employers' health care costs. A hospital's package of services may include programs designed to help employers develop incentives for employees to make more appropriate use of hospital emergency rooms, physicians' offices, and alternative providers. Hospitals and clinics are also changing their products and services to reduce costs. Most important, they are developing strategies for selling and promoting their new services and approaches to delivering health care.

In *Health Care Marketing Plans: From Strategy to Action,* Steven G. Hillestad and Eric N. Berkowitz describe the business opportunities available to clinics and hospitals. Then they show how providers can learn what their customers want and need, and how to successfully fill those needs. The authors save planners hundreds of hours of committee meetings by listing important questions that should be asked when planning a marketing strategy and milestones to check while the plan is being implemented. They not only provide questions and checklists but also a variety of strategies that will work in some business environments and not in others. The decisions about which questions to ask and strategies to adopt, of course, are left up to the readers.

This book fills a critical gap in the health care literature. It gives marketing managers and chief executive officers a workable way to decide what businesses they should be in and how to attack their marketing opportunities both responsibly and profitably. *Health Care Marketing Plans: From Strategy to Action* should be read by every clinic and hospital administrator, and it should be required reading for marketing students in both undergraduate and graduate courses in health care administration and public health administration.

Donald E. L. Johnson
Editor
MODERN HEALTHCARE
Chicago, Illinois

FOREWORD

During most of the past 100 years, the health care business in the United States has functioned using a fairly simple structural model. That was a decentralized, cottage industry system with a multitude of individual operators (physicians, hospitals, pharmacies, other services) offering a fairly homogenous type of service, differentiated mainly by their geographic distribution. After World War II, this model began to change—first slowly, but in the last decade with great acceleration and dynamism. Social policy, technology, scarcity of capital resources, and an increasing number of both physicians and health care facilities have worked to drive these changes. Today the health care business is being reshaped into centralized and well-structured organizations. These are designed to compete effectively and efficiently with other medical organizations in the marketplace. These organizations are rapidly sweeping away the old delivery model built around the cottage industry style.

Although competition is not new in the health care business, its style and expression in today's marketplace are quite different than they were in the past. The marketplace that is evolving is much more a buyers' market than health care workers have ever experienced in the past. It is populated by a diverse set of buyers. Some are large third-party payors or industries seeking a better price for big volumes of potential business. Some are individuals looking for a new product or greater product suitability (access, style, convenience). Still others seek a stronger position in negotiating the exchange and its associated attributes. The effective organizational competitors in that market are quickly recognizing that effective management systems are essential to function in this new market where consumers are ever more assertive and demanding.

The first job of management in the health care organization is to develop its agenda; its program; its organized response. These matters can no longer be left to chance, as was possible in earlier and more comfortable times when demand was limitless and resources bountiful. The plan of response in the future cannot be provider-oriented. It must be oriented to the needs and desires of health care consumers. The "doctor knows best" belief of the past is now being replaced by a realization that the health care consumer has needs, wants, and demands, which can profitably be addressed if the institution will pay heed to those desires.

The development of an organized plan focused on the health care consumer means a marketing approach to the planning and delivery of health care services. That will not be easy for many in health care because so much of the structure of health care was built around professional norms and desires. These were deeply internalized in the medical profession and in the organizational health care business as it has existed. There remains in the health care business a pervasive belief that the professionals should "prescribe" and the consumers should be "patient." At best many providers believe the problem is to "educate the patients." The authority of the provider is still felt to be a self-evident necessity by many. Nevertheless, the prototype organizations of the future are already visible in abundance. These are organizations that are emphasizing horizontal and vertical integration to accomplish both internal efficiency and marketplace adaptability. They are organizations that are concerned with access, convenience, price, and health as a positive characteristic of life rather than the absence of a negative characteristic. There are organizations that are rejecting the traditional separation of powers within the institution that left management and the medical staff in adversarial positions. There are organizations that are grouping the whole range of health care workers into teams that will make them adaptable to marketplace opportunity. There are organizations that are moving beyond the comfort and familiarity of the "corner grocery store" to the efficiency and enormously expanded effectiveness of the modern service establishment.

The next 10 years promise an extensive reorganization for the business of delivering health care services. Health care as a one-on-one process concerned only with the elimination of disease, carried out in a cottage industry, is passing away. It is in transition. It is becoming a service industry that must focus all the resources of a complex science and art upon the lifetime needs of a knowledgeable consumer. It is an ever more competitive business that requires the highest order of management and organizational effectiveness if success is to be forthcoming. It will be a business where the survivors understand their market and are responsive to it. It is to promote such discipline that this book was created.

David J. Ottensmeyer, M.D.
President
Lovelace Medical Foundation
Albuquerque, New Mexico

PREFACE

Health care is rapidly moving into the competitive age, which will see new patterns of delivery emerge as a competitive response to changing marketplace conditions. With these new conditions, marketing strategy will become critical.

Up to this point, strategy (when it existed in an organization) has been articulated in "the plan." While these plans look nice in the beautiful leather binder, they are often only partially successful.

An analysis of plans that have gone astray often reveals several key problems:

1. The plan is strategically and tactically weak.
2. The action portion of the plan is inappropriate or not detailed.
3. Health care organizations often make the mistaken assumption that their organization's intuitive sense of the marketplace can correctly anticipate consumer needs.

This book will show health care executives how to avoid the traditional mistakes and how to make marketing work for the organization. This book concentrates on the critical area of connecting the *proper selection* of a strategy to the *proper implementation* of that strategy. Another key feature of the book is the presentation, in one volume, of all the basic elements and decision topics that are essential to a marketing plan, but which, until now, have not been joined together. Therefore, a methodology is presented which shows the elements of a marketing program working in harmony from start to finish. By using a market-based approach to business planning, a higher level of success can be achieved.

We hope readers of this book will gain a new understanding of the challenge, potential, and role of health care marketing.

Steven G. Hillestad
Eric N. Berkowitz, Ph.D.

ACKNOWLEDGMENTS

This book is the result of input and support from many people. The foundation of the book is based on a number of experiences with physicians, executives, and managers with whom we have had the opportunity to consult, take part in seminars, and discuss how marketing can work in health care. The experiences gained with these people helped to provide the necessary insight from which the book was developed.

Special recognition must also be given to several other people. First, to Fairview Community Hospitals, and specifically, Carl Platou, president and chief executive officer of this innovative multiunit system. Mr. Platou was fully supportive of the time spent in the development of this project and the sharing of information contained in this book with the entire health care industry. Without Mr. Platou's interest and the availability of the creative environment which he cultivates at Fairview, this book probably would not have been written.

Gordon Johnson, president of Madison General Hospital in Madison, Wisconsin, is another leading health care executive who deserves special recognition. His organization was one of the first hospitals in the country to use marketing strategy and tactics to develop new ventures long before marketing was popular around the country. This experience was helpful in forming early recognition that marketing can work in health care.

A silent partner in this process was Helen Donnay. She watched us write draft chapters which she, in turn, edited, corrected, and typed only to see us change the material to such an extent that she had to start again. She coordinated typing, material preparation, and the problem of keeping an eye on all the pieces of the book. Helen, thanks for your help. Any final mistakes in this manuscript, however, are the fault of the authors.

Another individual who contributed to the project was Pamela Effertz, a co-worker at Fairview Community Hospitals. Her reading of the manuscript and exhibits resulted in greater clarity and accuracy. She also watched us putting the book together and offered her support while quietly wondering how it could be possible for the two of us to finish the task.

Several people offered critical comments regarding exhibits, manuscript, and conceptual ideas. These individuals include clients, students, and co-workers. We want to offer special recognition to Rolf Hanson, Rob Meyer, and Dottie Young for the critical review each offered. Thank you for your help.

While all these people provided valuable hours of support, the ultimate responsibility for the book rests with us. The opinions expressed here are ours and do not necessarily reflect the attitudes or opinions of the organizations for which we work.

To everyone involved in this book, thank you for your help, support, understanding, honesty, and humor.

S. G. H.
E. N. B.

▨ CONTENTS

CHAPTER 1

THE CHALLENGE OF A COMPETITIVE MARKETPLACE

Developing effective marketing plans is essential to any ongoing health care organization. This is not always easy because the environment in which medicine is practiced is undergoing change on several fronts. Thus, before the specific approaches to outlining marketing strategies are detailed, the macro changes that affect any strategy will be briefly highlighted. These changes come from:

Government.
Consumers.
Competitors.
Industry.

Health care is an attractive target for many regulators. Consumer insistence that health care is a right gives it important political impact. Also, the rising cost of health care makes regulatory review necessary in this area.

■ Regulatory Change

In 1981, about $287 billion was spent on health care—a 15 percent increase over the year before. About 43 percent of that total was provided by government sources.[1] Recent data suggest that the gross national product (GNP) accounted for by health care is in the neighborhood of 9.8 percent and still climbing. More alarming, however, is the fact that the cost for health care services, left unchecked, would more than double in the early 1990s. The federal government does not want the present system of health care to continue at this rate of increasing cost. Therefore, governments at both the federal and state level are currently looking at the possibility of implementing models of competition designed to make physicians and hospitals more price competitive.

One model causing interest in government became legal on July 1, 1982, in California. Under this plan, Medi-Cal patients get their care in a few, selected California hospitals with state contracts obtained through a price-competitive bidding process. No longer can Medi-Cal patients and their doctors choose locations for medical care. Instead, doctors use only hospitals that have contracts. This approach causes hospitals to compete intensely with one another, and the purchaser of care can now exercise some buying control regarding providers.

A variation of this theme was introduced in Minnesota in early 1983 by Blue Cross/Blue Shield. In it, contracts were signed with hospitals which, in some cases, had to provide discounts of 45 percent in order to be included. Other competitive models revolve around the elimination of such laws and regulations as government-mandated health planning.

Deregulation is the government buzzword for the 1980s. Although for several years health care providers complained of the strict regulatory controls, many of these same people will soon realize the impact of a less-regulated environment.

Recently deregulated industries, such as airlines and trucking, demonstrate how dramatically business practices can change. Previously in the airline industry, companies wishing to do business on specific routes had to apply for the equivalent of a certificate-of-need in these protected areas. Now any competitor can enter into new routes or existing territories, and it is generally felt that, because of the elimination of the certificate-of-need (CON) and the dramatic expansion of certain routes, many companies in the airline industry are in serious trouble. (Exhibit 1–1 shows the significant change in airline return on assets when deregulation occurred.) On the hospital side, administrators who were at first enamored with the concept of deregulation are now more thoughtful and concerned about what might happen in their own deregulated, price-competitive environment.

In essence, we can forecast first, that the government will change its approach to the purchase of health care services including prospective payments using Diagnostic Related Groups (DRGs) in order to control runaway costs. Second, the elimination of regulation, a seemingly positive change, may in fact, bring a competitive onslaught that health care people could not have foreseen.

---

[1]Peat, Marwick, Mitchell & Co., *Management Focus,* (March/April 1983), p. 21.

EXHIBIT 1–1
Return on Assets in the Airline Industry Before and After Deregulation

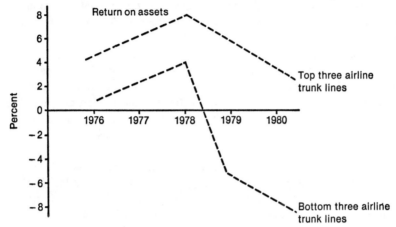

Note: "Competitive Deregulation" occurred in 1978.
Source: Louden & Company. Teri Louden, President, Chicago, Ill. Used by permission
© 1983.

■ The Consumer

The changing attitudes and habits of the modern-day consumer are not only interesting topics, but also causes for concern as they force us to reconsider the practice of medicine in the 1980s. The new consumer is well-educated, earns more money than ever before, and is an independent thinker, who is concerned about brand names and interested in switching brands to obtain better quality. He often gets second opinions, does things for himself, and is generally self-reliant.

While other countries are seeing an increase in population, the United States is undergoing a slowdown in population growth. The declining birthrate is a concern for some industries; an opportunity for others. It causes problems for those companies involved in children's toys, clothes, furniture and food. Johnson & Johnson has responded by trying to interest adults in using its baby powder and shampoo. Burger King has added a salad bar to attract older markets. Abbott Laboratories has added a geriatric food line to complement its line of infant formulas.[2] The low birthrate also presents problems for pediatricians, but opportunities for other specialists. In the years ahead, the over-65 age group will show a large rate of growth, increasing by at least 23 million Americans and perhaps as many as 32 million by the year 2000. This expected increase foretells a burgeoning demand for retirement homes and communities, campers, quiet forms of recreation (fishing, golf), single-portion food packaging, and such medical

---

[2]Philip Kotler, *Marketing Management* (Englewood Cliffs, N.J.: Prentice-Hall, 1980), p. 104.

goods and services as medicine, eyeglasses, canes, hearing aids, and convalescent homes. The growth of this group will also mean more conservative politics, new demands by senior citizens for the right to protect their standard of living, and a slowdown in the adoption of diverse cultural ideas.[3]

The American ideal of the two-child, two-car suburban family, which provided great marketing opportunity in the post-World War II period, is changing. Working women now constitute a large market for better clothing, child day care, home cleaning services, frozen dinners, and evening clinic hours. As people's incomes and lifestyles change further, we can expect pronounced shifts in the demands for different categories of goods and services.

In general, the market today is a fickle one, skeptical and independent. It is willing to change loyalties quickly, shop options, and is less likely to develop long-term relationships. A proprietary study conducted for one hospital revealed that 18.2 percent of the people surveyed in a major metropolitan area were considering changing their physicians.

Mom and Dad were more likely to have pie and coffee at the local café, vacation at a family-owned resort, buy cars year after year from the same neighborhood dealer, shop for groceries at the local, independently owned grocery store (saying "hello" to the owner behind the check-out counter), buy hardware from the local hardware store because they trusted the owner's knowledge and knew his kids, and see the family physician known for years and years. The new generation of consumers is more likely to have breakfast at McDonald's, vacation at a Marriott Resort, buy milk at Tom Thumb, buy hardware at Sears, and belong to an HMO. In these cases, the important factor in the consumer's mind is not the personal relationship, but instead, the perception of consistency, convenience, price, and brand image. In fact, studies are beginning to show consumers saying they play a major role in hospital selection, and physicians corroborate this evaluation.

What does this type of market mean for the health care community? One resounding impact might be the new concept of individuals taking care of themselves; not relying on third parties and not simply accepting therapies, consults, prescriptions, and advice. In fact, self-help medical care seems to be the "blossoming of America's entrepreneurial movement," to use a phrase of John Naisbitt's from his book, *Megatrends—Ten New Directions Transforming Our Lives*.[4] In this book, Naisbitt examines how so-called health nuts of the early 1970s have been transformed into mainstream consumers. Think of how jogging has grown from a cult to a mass movement.

At least 100 million Americans are now exercising in some way,

---

[3]Ibid., p. 105.

[4]John Naisbitt, *Megatrends—Ten New Directions Transforming Our Lives* (New York: Warner Books, 1982), p. 133.

whereas in 1960 only about one quarter of the population did. Fat intake has been reduced by 20 percent. Smoking among men is down 28 percent since 1965. People have switched from hard liquor to wine, and in 1980, for the first time, wine consumption outpaced that of hard liquor. The number of health food stores increased from 1,200 in 1968 to more than 6,000 in 1978. In the same period, health food sales went from $170 million to $1.6 billion. Two hundred of the Fortune 500 companies belong to the business group on health, and more than 500 companies across the United States have full-time fitness directors. Along with the individual responsibility people are taking for their health, we are also seeing tremendous expansion in the self-help medical movement. Americans no longer run to a doctor for every ailment.

In New York, residents can send $1 to the American Cancer Society and receive a bowel cancer test kit. It is now possible to monitor blood pressure at home or test for pregnancy, diabetes, or infection. In 1981, home health care was a $3.1 billion dollar business, up from $500 million 10 years earlier. One large New York market research house indicates that sales in the home health care market will be at least $10 billion by the 1990s.[5]

The American Medical Association has fashioned an interesting response to the type of consumer now in the marketplace. The AMA family health guide, published in the fall of 1982, is scheduled to be offered as a Book-of-the-Month Club feature selection. The feature of the book that is, perhaps, most startling to the medical care community is also most attractive to the self-help consumer. The book contains a number of decision trees which allow the consumer to analyze his symptoms through a set of detailed, yet very easy-to-follow instructions. The consumer starts with a basic symptom and is led to a series of possible conclusions, such as the need to see a physician or the suggestion that self-care is sufficient.[6] While no physician wants needless visits from patients, or unnecessary work, many suggestions provided in the guidebook represent advice that used to be given by physicians in their offices. How are these lost patient visits made up?

In addition, we are finding that consumers, when in need of a physician's services, are now more than ever, willing to seek alternatives to traditional forms of care. A *New York Times* survey indicated that patients are more willing to be treated by assistants rather than by a physician and to go to clinics where a doctor is immediately available instead of waiting for their own private doctor.[7] These findings mirror consumer behavior in the marketplace. Personal relationships, whether in the marketplace or in the doctor's office, seem to be less important than the right brand and the

---

[5]The Non-Institutional Senior Market for Healthcare Products and Services (New York: Frost & Sullivan, 1982).

[6]Jeffrey Kunz, M.D., ed., *The American Medical Association Family Health Guide* (New York: Random House, 1982).

[7]Robert Reinhold, "Majority in Survey on Healthcare Open to Changes to Cut Costs," *New York Times,* March 29, 1982.

convenience. For some physicians, this kind of consumer activity represents opportunity, but for others, it means fewer patients.

An article in *Psychology Today* reported results of a poll of 25,000 of the magazine's rather up-scale readers.[8] Findings showed several areas of concern about their doctors. Of readers who had visited a physician in the past year, 49 percent complained about the waiting time in the doctor's office. Another 36 percent complained about being charged too much, and 25 percent of the respondents felt a condescending or uncaring attitude was displayed by the doctor. Again, it would seem that the consumer in the physician's office is not unlike the consumer exercising buying power in the marketplace at large. He is more critical, more independent, more willing to search out alternatives, and less tolerant of delays.

As more health care alternatives are provided, the dissatisfied patient can change providers with greater ease. Several studies have revealed the size of this skeptical consumer segment. In a typical urban area, over 30 percent of a given population claims they do not have or do not care to have a physician.[9] When probed further, the vast majority of these consumers could find no difference in quality between an HMO and a private arrangement. They also have a great willingness to explore options that involve convenience at a reasonable cost. As market plans are developed, recognition of this changing consumer is essential. Plans developed to meet consumer needs even five years ago may not reflect the patient with today's attitudes and values.

It is reasonable to suggest that the medical care consumer of tomorrow will second-guess judgments, be more willing to obtain second opinions, be likely to search for fresh alternatives, be more interested in convenience, and will not necessarily cherish or understand the meaning of or need for personal medical care relationships (except possibly for those cases when long-term chronic care or crisis intervention is required).

In some respects, medicine has not actively done much to offset this trend. For example, the medical profession, by and large, has treated industrial medicine cases with distaste, as demonstrated by slow follow-up, paperwork errors, and a general lack of interest in this area. Even the specialty of occupational medicine has been viewed as second-class by some. As a result, industry has sought out better, more reliable service, and doctors are now beginning to recognize this area as a hot, new market.

Chemical dependency is another area that has been unattractive to physicians. It is also now a hot market—a market being served by corporations that see opportunities because physicians haven't responded.

A third area that has been neglected is that of nonemergent emergency

---

[8]Carin Rubenstein, "Wellness is All," *Psychology Today*, October 1982, p. 37.

[9]Data gathered through unpublished market research conducted in metropolitan areas.

care. How many meetings are held in hospitals by the staff to discuss the call list, the unassigned patient, and whether or not the physician on call needs to come in at 11 p.m. for upper respiratory complaints? For years most doctors hated this area, but today it is one that doctors are beginning to fight over, in order to grab the business. Again, here is a burgeoning market, and one into which entrepreneurial companies and physicians are moving, quickly and aggressively.

■ Physicians Are Changing

The consumer and the government are not the only factors causing change in the health care environment. The next few years will see an astounding growth in the number of physicians (estimated to increase 79 percent between 1970 and 1990).[10] Traditional medical practices can be expected to change, and dramatic growth in new group practices has already been reported.

A new type of physician is also emerging. The bright, young, hardworking physician does not want to be run over by the supply of competing physicians in the marketplace. Therefore, many of these physicians are becoming highly entrepreneurial—changing practice patterns, joining HMOs, becoming competitive, acting in a business environment, applying business skills to a clinical setting, and becoming aggressive—merely in order to survive.

Physicians who are pursuing the establishment of chains of clinics across the United States are an example of this entrepreneurial spirit which is intensified not only by a large supply of physicians, but also by the fact that these physicians believe that the changing consumer marketplace will respond. The result may be the establishment of urgent care centers, occupational medicine clinics, or a range of other services that many physicians traditionally would not or could not provide.

The economics of medicine has heightened the entrepreneurial and competitive spirit of many physicians. *Medical Economics* recently reported on a survey of physicians that indicated a drop in the median number of weekly patient visits between 1978 and 1982 of 126 visits to 108 visits, or about a 20 percent decline.[11] Within the last two years, independent research has indicated a substantial decline in appointment backlog, so that most patients can now easily see a doctor within days, as opposed to weeks, for services such as physical exams. *Medical Economics* data corroborate this finding by noting that the percent of physicians who indicated they were at

---

[10]Jeffrey Goldsmith, *Can Hospitals Survive?* (Homewood, Ill.: Dow Jones-Irwin, 1981), p. 29.

[11]Meriam Kirchner, "Where Have All the Patients Gone?" *Medical Economics,* Dec. 20, 1982, p. 151.

8

full capacity dropped from 69 percent in 1978 to 51 percent in the 1982 study.[12] These changes in demand require a reevaluation of physician practice patterns.

For example, evening hours are becoming a common tool used to attract or maintain patient volume. With the vast increase in two-income households and with women consuming a large share of medical service, the availability to evening hours is a natural market response. Other responses include clinics located in shopping malls and drive-in pediatric clinics. In some cities, doctors are organized strictly for the purpose of making house calls. One writer recently suggested that the house call is one of the routine services coming back as a competitive response by physicians trying to hold on to their oftentimes dwindling practices.[13] These shrinking practices are occurring because there are more physicians coming into the market and providing consumers with more alternatives.

These changes often represent strategic marketing warfare between physicians. This movement isn't necessarily sweeping the country or becoming a national phenomenon, but as the environment changes, marketing warfare can be expected among all parties in the health care scene—government, hospitals, physicians, and corporations.

■ The Changing Hospital Environment

It's not possible to discuss health care competition without evaluating the hospital environment. In most communities, hospitals are at a critical stage in their existence. Profits have been squeezed dramatically, lengths of stay are down, numbers of patients are down, negative press is increasing, capital requirements are skyrocketing, and generally, the business future is bleak.

The difficulties noted here are causing fundamental changes in the hospital. Now, what used to be characterized as "the hospital" or "community hospital" is more likely to be called "the hospital industry." By the end of 1982, 773 hospitals were run by for-profit hospital chains, the largest of which is Hospital Corporation of America (HCA). HCA has 306 hospitals, gross revenues of $2.9 billion and a net income of $171 million. Thirteen years ago, HCA did not exist. Wall Street will no doubt continue to watch this proprietary industry carefully as growth and profits skyrocket.[14]

In 1982, 1,740 hospitals were owned by, leased and managed by, or participated in hospital systems.[15] These systems grew out of two perceived needs. First, management systems believe their size allows better management and overall strategy development execution. Second, these organiza-

---

[12]Ibid.

[13]Jeffrey Goldsmith, interview on the Today Show, NBC–TV, February 25, 1982.

[14]Donald Johnson, "Multi Units Are Ready to Boost Market Share," *Modern Healthcare,* May 1983, p. 89.

[15]*Hospital Statistics, 1982 Edition* (Chicago: American Hospital Association), p. 15.

tions feel that their approach allows for better management of capital. At present, about 30 percent of hospitals are part of a chain or system. Many of the hospitals that have chosen this route recognized that the core business of the traditional hospital was in trouble. These hospitals have decided to examine alternative methods of organization and business definition. Several excellent examples of the alternatives which may cause the hospital's core business to decline have been developed by Jeffrey Goldsmith.[16]

EXHIBIT 1–2
Competitive Alternatives to Hospital Care

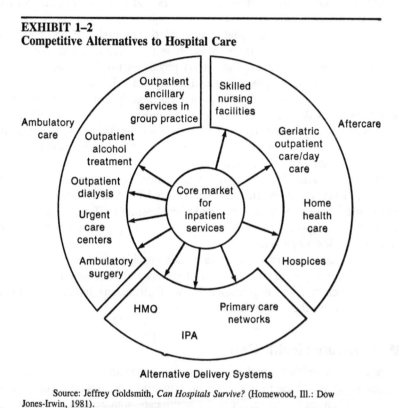

Alternative Delivery Systems

Source: Jeffrey Goldsmith, *Can Hospitals Survive?* (Homewood, Ill.: Dow Jones-Irwin, 1981).

Exhibit 1–2 indicates that services ranging from home health care to ambulatory surgery to dialysis centers are all viable alternatives to the increasingly expensive hospital. In general, the core business for the hospital is in serious jeopardy. This reality is causing tremendous competition and conflict between one hospital and another, as well as between hospitals and physicians.

---

[16]Goldsmith, *Can Hospitals Survive?* p. 16.

Physicians are becoming increasingly concerned about the intrusion of hospitals into the actual practice of medicine. Hospitals, on the other hand, are concerned about their bread and butter since business is being eroded by the opening of surgery centers, urgent care centers, and diagnostic centers that are often owned by physicians. Combined, these three alternatives alone can eliminate 50 percent of a typical hospital's business. This, in effect, creates a "hospital without walls," owned by physicians. Therefore, hospitals are trying to respond by fostering new services, trying to find new physicians, and getting into businesses or services that physicians often feel are out of the bounds of the hospital.

At the same time, hospitals recognize the necessity of being closely attuned to the physician's needs. Many hospitals have invested in doctors' office buildings in an attempt to attract physician loyalty. Space in these buildings is provided to physicians under very attractive terms.

Hospitals are also beginning to market directly to the consumer. Research indicates that although doctors bring most cases to the hospital, numerous patients come directly to the hospital for care. This fact has led many hospitals to attempt to increase their visibility in hopes of establishing a strong consumer preference. Some hospitals, such as those under Hospital Corporation of America, are trying a guaranteed satisfaction, money-back program. Even more patients can be attracted through insurance carriers, which direct volume to approved doctors and hospitals. Thus, hospitals have begun to work more closely with new third-party payment alternatives in spite of physician opposition.

The marketing strategies of health care providers must change because hospitals have begun to change. New programs and increased awareness of markets other than those generated by staff physicians indicate a greater agressiveness by these organizations.

■ Corporate Health Care

Another important factor is the interest that corporations have in health care. On one hand, health care is viewed as an attractive business opportunity. For example, Humana is a large, for-profit health care organization, listed on the New York Stock Exchange. Indications are that Humana is interested in moving rather quickly into the extended office hours business, which includes what is called the "urgent care" concept.[17] Currently, Humana expects to operate 100 "Med First" clinics and is considering up to 500, which, when tied together, would become a national brand for medical care. This urgent care concept is one of the fastest-moving trends seen in health care today, and the success of this method of care may be directly related to capital spending. In mid-1983, one expert estimated that about 1.5 units are

---

[17]Howard Eisenberg, "The Competition You'll Face in 1983," *Medical Economics*, Jan. 10, 1983, p. 242.

opening each day in the United States. This is likely to create a tremendous amount of competition.

In essence, the urgent care center is a clinic interested in episodic cases, including care for patients who do not wish to have a personal physician. The clinics operate from approximately 8 A.M. to 11 P.M. and do not require scheduled appointments. These organizations cater to patients who typically would have gone to a hospital emergency room for care, or would have tried to set up an episodic visit with a physician. Located in shopping centers, the clinics use the franchise approach. Closely structured, they are fast, clean, convenient, and apparently provide very satisfactory care. It is estimated that these centers can take from 40 to 50 percent of all patients away from hospital emergency rooms and a similar number away from doctors' offices.

Developers of national chains of free-standing emergency care centers, ambulatory surgical centers, industrial medicine clinics, and extended-hour physicians' offices are planning to add dozens of units in the next few years.

The importance of this concept is that it comes from within the medical establishment or, at least, from within the medical community. It involves those entrepreneurial physicians, moving into many communities across the United States, who are interested in leading consumers away from "Mom and Pop" medical practices to franchised care centers. Corporate chain systems have already entered the areas of restaurants, hotels, retail stores, and legal and accounting services. Now they are beginning to transform traditional methods of medical care in this country.

■ Technology

Technology is also causing concern for the health care industry, as technology-driven industries are most susceptible to change. Within a short period of time, a hospital's technical advantage can be eliminated as competing hospitals purchase the newest generation of particular diagnostic equipment.

Likewise, technological innovations increasingly shift inpatient procedures to outpatient activities, or even eliminate some procedures totally. Will laser surgery make eye work largely outpatient in nature? Will semiconductors alter cardiac pacemaker care? Will new methods such as the auto suture stapling technique reduce length of hospital stay? Will nuclear magnetic resonance (NMR) technology cause the CT scan to become outdated? Will mobile scanning companies such as Medi Q of California change hospital and clinic referral patterns? And, whereas over 2,300 companies manufacture medical equipment, will the eight which control over 50 percent of all shipments try to leverage the industry?

Recognizing the technological impact on health care means that no provider is protected from change beyond its control. The marketplace must be examined for new opportunities as a safeguard against the technological elimination of anyone's core businesses. (Where are TB hospitals today?)

■ Payment Systems

For years, government, business, and consumers have complained about health care costs. Only recently, however, have we started to see substantial attempts to seek solutions, with alternative systems being tested, tried, and legislated.

Government is moving from a retrospective, fee-for-service system to a prospective, package-price approach. For the first time, purchasers of care will be able to compare prices, and providers will be able to promote their own price advantages through DRG systems. Other pricing strategies are being explored, for example, the Preferred Provider Organization (PPO), which is largely a discount pricing strategy focused on finding new patient volume.

Further, a recently reported Rand study of 7,700 consumers found that if employers pay 100 percent of the health care costs, expenditures are likely to be 50 percent more than they are when employees pay 95 percent of the first $1,000 of medical bills.[18] Shifting more risk to consumers is a likely payment change for many corporations and insurance companies. Other innovative methods, such as insurance company rebates to patients who leave the hospital one or two days early and cash to employees who find and correct errors in medical bills, are becoming more common.

HMOs also continue to grow. From 1981 to 1982, the number of HMOs grew from 243 to 265 plans or a 9 percent increase.[19] Although it is not clear if such growth will continue, it is recognized that HMOs do have the power to draw patients, physicians, and business investors—causing the private, fee-for-service community more reason for concern.

■ Corporate Concern

The major influence on the future plans of health care providers may be the private corporation. In recent years, companies have experienced an average yearly increase of 12 percent in health care costs. Through most of the 1970s, corporations viewed health care as a necessary overhead expense, similar to other fixed costs. In recent years, however, the attitude toward health care cost has changed. Instead of being seen as fixed costs, these expenditures are now being viewed as controllable expenses. As they do with costs for distribution, sales, or advertising, companies are examining ways to control these rising health care charges.

The corporate response to increasing health care expenses has taken several forms. Many organizations have begun to offer the HMO option. Groups such as the National Association of Employers for Health Maintenance Organizations (NAEHMO) have been developed by industry to aid in the HMO offering decision. Study has shown that companies belonging to

---

[18]Peat, Marwick, *Management Focus*, p. 17.

[19]"HMOs Increase 9 Percent in 1982," *Hospitals*, April 16, 1983, p. 19.

NAEHMO have higher HMO corporate penetration than non-NAEHMO members.[20]

Prepaid health care is only one option being pursued by companies. Other alternatives have been developed to monitor changes in the fee-for-service sector. Some organizations have joined business coalitions to monitor health care costs in their areas. Another response has been in the form of a private review program. Employees who are under review may see their regular physician. However, decisions on hospitalization must receive approval from the review office. This approach is a more aggressive attempt to watch costs by health care providers.

The greatest impact on existing health care providers from corporations may not be in the form of cost-containment efforts. Rather, some corporations may see health care as an area of strong opportunity. Consider organizations such as Sears. This company has strong name recognition, a positive identity, multiple sites, and its own credit system. Envision the Sears Primary Care Center. When you enter, you give your credit card to the receptionist. Your medical records appear. The doctor is 20 minutes behind schedule. The receptionist gives you a paging beeper and invites you to go shopping. When the doctor is within five minutes of seeing you, the pager will beep. As part of the Sears guarantee, if the doctor is more than 45 minutes late, you get a $3 coupon to apply to your charge balance or next Sears purchase.

Think about the Sears HMO plan. Charge your premium. When you travel, there is always a Sears store nearby. Sears will then approach the local hospital, or selected specialty care providers, for per capita payments. Unlikely? Sears and People's Drug publish medical supply catalogs. Why not retail medicine or dentistry on the corporate chain scale? Johnson & Johnson is a trusted name so why shouldn't it move more directly into HMOs, clinic development, or home health care?

Companies, the traditional payors of health care bills, have reexamined their role. Some private organizations are seeing an aging market as a potentially profitable revenue base. Future marketing plans by existing health care organizations must recognize this more active, potentially competitive participant, the corporation.

So what does all this activity mean? It means change. It means that success in health care is no longer guaranteed. It means a more difficult, businesslike climate where strategy becomes important. As a result, hospitals, doctors, and other health care businesses will need to develop a strategic mind set, selecting among alternative courses of action based on logic, clinical sense, and market sense. Therefore, the market plan will become the foundation on which strategic decisions are made and action plans implemented.

---

[20]Richard C. Becherer and Lawrence M. Richard, "Study Says Most Offer HMOs, Add Alcohol Plan," *Business Insurance*, Oct. 2, 1978, p. 16.

▨ CHAPTER 2

STRATEGY DEVELOPMENT AND THE STRATEGIC MINDSET

The ultimate purpose of any market plan is to develop effective strategy that will be successful in helping an organization realize its objectives. Broadly speaking, the term "strategy" implies the development of plans to reach a goal. As this definition indicates, the process of market plan development used in this book will be goal oriented.

The notion of strategizing to attain a goal is useful in business, athletics, personal financial planning, and a variety of other activities. However, the use of strategy in a business environment takes on a special interpretation as outlined by Bruce Henderson, chairman of the Boston Consulting Group. "Any useful strategy must include a means of upsetting the competitive equilibrium and reestablishing it again on a more favorable basis."[1] The foundation for Henderson's statement is the assumption that the organization developing a strategy wishes to grow. Of course, one should also assume that the other organizations competing in the same territory or service also wish to grow. Therefore, there are multiple organizations attempting to reach the same potential end point (growth). It is thus often necessary for the successful organization to change the competitive situation and attempt to dominate, using strategies which are more favorable to its own goals.

Developing useful strategy includes several important steps. First is the

---

[1]Bruce Henderson, *Henderson on Corporate Strategy* (Cambridge, Mass.: Abt Books, 1979), p. 3.

need to "upset the competitive equilibrium." Within most communities there exists a competitive equilibrium among hospitals, clinics, insurance carriers, and other health-related businesses, often with dominance by one hospital or large medical clinic. Many physicians consider these organizations members of a medical fraternity. This is to say that while the physicians and/or hospitals may be competitive with one another, this competition is often limited to exclude the use of overt and aggressive competitive strategy.

Because of the recognition of the medical fraternity, groups are often reluctant to consider the establishment of clinics outside of the "territory." For the same reason, hospitals are often averse to making major moves. In order for useful strategy to occur, however, it is necessary for all physicians and health-related executives to realize the need to upset the competitive equilibrium.

Second, consider "reestablishing it (equilibrium) again on a more favorable basis." This phrase refers to the development of strategy along the lines of new concepts, ideas, and product offerings, or serving markets that have not been thought of before or thought to be worthwhile. It is within this area that health care innovation can be expected. In other words, reestablishing on a more favorable basis may mean offering a new service, such as an urgent care center to successfully compete against the traditional hospital emergency room. This is an example of the advantage a lower-cost service has over the hospital emergency room. A retaliatory response from the hospital is difficult.

Once the organization begins to develop a sense of what the term strategy means and has an opportunity to begin to develop related marketing plans, it becomes clear that the market plans and the strategy are not passive in nature. These concepts are appropriate for a competitive environment. It is also quite obvious that these terms are action oriented. Competitive actions are necessary for achieving organizational goals.

■ Steps for Strategy Development

How does an organization start the process of developing a new strategy? Four steps have been suggested: (1) defining the area of business involved; (2) identifying competitors; (3) identifying differences among competitors; and (4) forecasting environmental change.[2]

These steps refer to the generation of information which can help the organization make alternative decisions. In Chapter 5 of this book an extensive analysis of the methods used to uncover the necessary data, plus questions which need to be asked in order to develop a market plan, are presented.

---

[2]Ibid., p. 18.

Once the data base has been developed, it is possible to begin selecting among alternative courses of action. The transition from data analysis to the selection of alternative action courses typically involves hundreds of separate decisions. These involve questions of which services to offer, which markets to serve, how to provide the services (i.e., centralized or de-centralized), which pricing strategies to use for different markets, services, and market-place conditions, and what the promotional strategies should be.

For example, a penetration strategy would consist of introducing a new service, such as wellness, at a low cost. The purpose of this strategy would be to maintain a broad-based market to assist in: (1) avoiding competitive entry by others, and (2) introducing the market to this new service in order to gain a large and lasting market share.

Another strategy option commonly used in marketing is a skim-pricing strategy, in which a new product or service is offered at a high price only to selected market segments. This method is used to recover investment or to gain marketplace status with the program. Often, as new competitors enter, prices are lowered. This is a strategy commonly used for high fashion clothing and technical items, such as digital watches and pocket calculators. It is also a strategy which can be employed in the health care environment. A skim-pricing strategy may be appropriate for the executive segment of the wellness market. After reaching the desired market share, the service can be broadened to include other segments at a more reasonable price.

Push or pull strategies are also common. The pull strategy consists of promoting to the customer with the hope that the customer will recommend the hospital or referral center. For example, promotion directly to the customers for a cardiology service would be based on the notion that when an individuals visits the family doctor and needs a stress EKG, he would ask to be referred to a particular hospital for the examination.

The push strategy, on the other hand, would have the hospital concentrate on promoting to the referral source, such as the physician. For example, when the patient goes to a family physician and is in need of a stress EKG, the physician would attempt to push the patient toward the cardiology unit that had been promoted to the doctor. This approach has been the most common with hospitals and referral clinics. Underlying this strategy is the belief that the primary care physician has the greatest influence on where the consumer gets care because the consumer will go wherever the family doctor suggests. Yet, as noted in Chapter 1, as more patients take a direct role in where they obtain their medical care, traditional strategies must be reexamined.

The preceding discussion of four marketing strategies indicates the wide degree of options availbale as one attempts to establish a competitive position. Virtually hundreds of other strategy options are also available. Therefore, the key is to develop the most appropriate information base possible to assist in determining which option has the greatest likelihood of success.

■ The Possibility of Failure

Frequently, organizations that move through a strategizing process to develop a plan, end up experiencing failure. Usually this failure is the result of: (1) errors in analyzing the data; (2) failure to gather appropriate data in the first place; (3) lack of specific objectives; or (4) failure to tie in the appropriate tactics. Stated another way, failure may be caused by a lack of tying strategy to action tactics.

Analysis of market plans, more common in hospitals than clinics, often lacks such data as information on consumers, referring physicians, and competitive pricing strategies. These oversights often lead to failure. This book outlines the data necessary to derive strategic option decisions.

Another source of failure is a lack of specific objectives and the logical tactics necessary to meet those objectives. Again, this book will explain the correct progression from gathering information to establishing firm objectives to developing the appropriate tactics.

In a recent article, Gordon Greenley documented how marketing planning fails in industry.[3] Based on a profile of 40 United Kingdom companies stratified by product groups, sales, and employees, 29 percent of the companies did not have specific product sales objectives. Thirty-two percent of the companies did not have marketing plan objectives on market sales. Many companies, both in and outside of health care, fail to set targeted objectives that would provide control and evaluation of ultimate success or failure. For strategy to be successful, market segments must be identified, and the appropriate strategy outlined for each group. An objective of this book is to provide necessary detail to assist health care organizations in addressing relevant market questions, establish workable objectives, and develop tactics that meet those objectives. In this way, the potential of the marketing function can be fully used.

Up to this point, strategy has been discussed within the broader context of general management. While this macro perspective is important, strategy must be viewed as a concept which is inherent in all levels of marketing plans. Strategy is important in setting the mission of the business, the marketing goals, the target market, and tactical option specification.

The concept of strategy as it relates to the mission of the health care business can be plotted on a continuum from narrow focus to broad focus as outlined in Exhibit 2–1. In Exhibit 2–1 the determination of mission becomes a strategy decision since it provides the organization's direction, sets its tone, and becomes the basis of future investment actions. The process of setting a mission is discussed in detail in Chapter 4. The important strategy consideration at this point is to select a mission capable of offering the greatest potential success–in a competitive environment and within a reasonable degree of risk.

---

[3]Gordon Greenley, "Where Marketing Planning Fails," *Long Range Planning* 16, no. 1, p. 106, 1983.

EXHIBIT 2–1
Strategic Mission Options

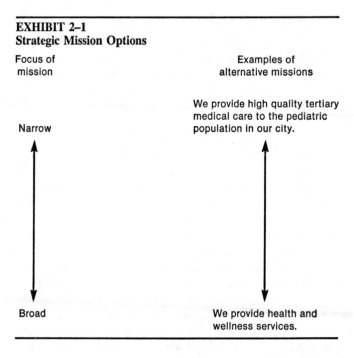

Focus of
mission

Examples of
alternative missions

Narrow

We provide high quality tertiary
medical care to the pediatric
population in our city.

Broad

We provide health and
wellness services.

Strategy is also important in selecting specific marketing options. Again, alternative courses of action are available and depend on the mission selected. Different outcomes occur as a function of this interaction. Exhibit 2–2 could involve a marketing goal strategy that seeks to get as many people as possible to try a new clinic in a one-year period, regardless of net income. An alternative strategy might be to maximize profitability without regard to total marketplace knowledge of the clinic.

Selection of one option over another is often difficult. However, it is necessary to select among alternative strategies in the goal-setting process because *it is not possible to maximize all possible marketing goal options at the same time.* One potential marketing goal option may be in conflict with a second alternative. For example, the goal of rapid gain in market share is in conflict with high immediate return on investment. Acquiring rapid growth in market share is expensive and often limits short-term profitability. Therefore, strategy is employed to weigh the alternative courses of action and to aid in the selection of the best alternatives. Chapters 4 and 5 help determine what conditions warrant various marketing goals.

As the marketing planning process moves from general to more specific action steps, strategy continues to play an important role. Exhibit 2–3 indicates different target markets by age. Marketing is based on the principle of effective strategy selection and should be oriented to defined market segments. For example, a pediatric practice does not serve all people but

EXHIBIT 2–2
Mission—Marketing Option Interaction

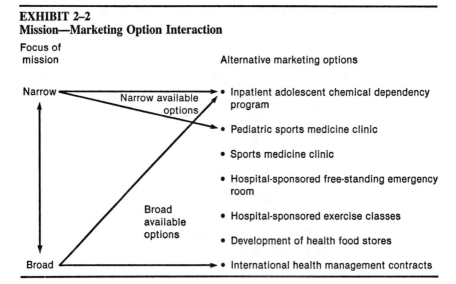

Focus of
mission   Alternative marketing options

Narrow   Narrow available   • Inpatient adolescent chemical dependency
                       options   program

                                                       • Pediatric sports medicine clinic

                                                       • Sports medicine clinic

                                                       • Hospital-sponsored free-standing emergency
                                                         room

                       Broad   • Hospital-sponsored exercise classes
                       available
                       options   • Development of health food stores

Broad   • International health management contracts

focuses on children and their parents. The strategy question involves selecting those target markets which: (a) have needs you can assist with and (b)
provide opportunity for success. Target markets in Exhibit 2–3 could be
young or old, middle income, suburban, women, upscale buyers, or a variety
of other descriptions.

It is again apparent that strategy is important in selecting target markets. A business can't concentrate on all markets; a clinic can't offer a full
range of health care services to all people. Therefore, choices must be made.
Strategic decisions must choose among alternative target markets based on
which market segments are most likely to assist in reaching the mission and

EXHIBIT 2–3
Target Market Focus

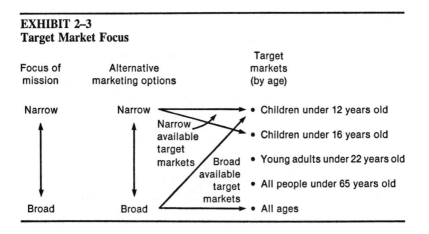

                                                       Target
Focus of   Alternative   markets
mission   marketing options   (by age)

Narrow   Narrow   • Children under 12 years old
                         Narrow
                         available   • Children under 16 years old
                         target
                         markets   Broad   • Young adults under 22 years old
                                         available
                                         target   • All people under 65 years old
                                         markets
Broad   Broad   • All ages

20

the marketing goals. These goals represent strategic alternatives selected earlier in the process. Chapters 4 and 5 will provide tools to help make these determinations.

The specific actions or tactics used to implement the marketing plan also involve strategy. Decisions at this level include product design, advertising, and pricing. Within each of these general areas, a variety of strategic alternatives are available. Action plans must be consistent with earlier strategic objectives.

For example, if a hotel set a marketing objective of expanding its share of the market among tourists over 65 years of age, logical action tactics would need to be developed to support this goal. These tactics might include discounts for seniors who are members of the American Association of Retired Persons (AARP), training front desk staff to speak up clearly, providing rooms that are close to hotel facilities, printing hotel information in a large type to make reading easier, menus that include plenty of poultry, fish, and fresh fruit, compact refrigerators in rooms to keep favorite light snacks and medicines, extra blankets, slip-proof materials in bathrooms, and the use of advertising strategies involving newspapers, magazines, and TV programs attractive to seniors.

All of these tactics represent logical strategy to support decisions made earlier in the plan. Exhibit 2–4 shows the several areas in which strategy, a key element throughout the entire process, is used in the development of marketing plans.

It is apparent that many strategy combinations are possible. This book focuses on helping health care organizations analyze their business and specify strategic decisions based on logical courses of action.

EXHIBIT 2–4
Alternative Marketing Tactics

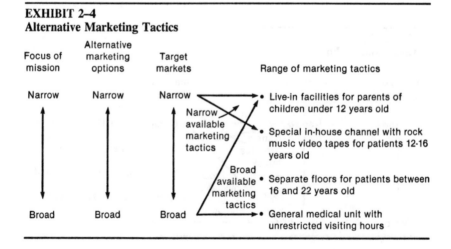

■ Developing the "Strategic Mind Set"

Before beginning the process of strategy development and ultimately the production of a market plan, an appropriate atmosphere within the organization is needed. This atmosphere is called "the strategic mind set." This phrase refers to a number of factors that must be in place and understood by all parties concerned in order for effective strategy development to occur. They include the attitudes of the key participants, as well as the understanding of some basic concepts of marketing and strategy development. Each element of the strategic mind set is reviewed in the following pages.

Services Cannot Remain Static; Change Is Inevitable

Many examples of products, goods, and services can be discussed to analyze the fact that today's successes can end up in moth balls tomorrow. The marketplace is constantly changing, and its needs and desires are dynamic. Technology is causing products to become obsolete at an ever-quickening rate.

Organizations that take a very narrow view of their product may miss opportunities for growth in tomorrow's market, while those that resist change may find themselves with no market to serve. Tuberculosis hospitals, hula hoops, and slide rulers are examples of products and services that are no longer needed or wanted by the modern consumer. This same concern pertains to hospitals and clinics in several services. The emergency room may be, in large part, replaced by urgent care clinics. The individual, personal physician is being replaced by the group practice, and the group practice may be replaced in many cases by a nationwide clinic organization. The most dangerous statement in developing strategy is, "We've been doing it this way for 30 years, and there's no reason to change." Physicians, hospitals, and businesses must dare to create a vision for tomorrow with change as a fundamental ingredient.

There Is Often a Better Way and Often the Competition Will Find It

Product and service innovation is a cornerstone of American business as well as of medicine. Today, innovations from business and medicine are coming together, often resulting in a better way. These positive steps have taken the form of improved approaches to organizing practices, better ways of paying for services, better technology to help patients stay out of the hospital, and, to the consumer, better ways of getting treatment through clinics in shopping malls, evening hours, and family billing plans.

As a result, when individuals within an organization sit down to develop strategy, they should not think that they have a lock on the best hospital, the best clinic, the best location, or the best physicians. These can become dangerous assumptions.

The Marketplace Has a Decision-Making Role in Helping to Direct the Future Course of a Business

This concept is often one of the most difficult to impress upon professionals who take daily responsibility for decisions on behalf of their patients. It is correct and appropriate that individuals in a professional capacity, such as physicians, assume such responsibility, but there are numerous occasions when patients should have the opportunity to make their own decisions regarding health care. From a marketing point of view, one of the most important elements in designing successful strategies is to ask consumers in the marketplace how they can be better served and what their needs are. Therefore, the marketplace is often in a position to assist in dictating office hours, fee ceilings, clinic locations, and a host of other elements. Basically, the types of decisions that consumers make regarding health care are the same types of decisions that health care professionals and other consumers make in the retail and commercial environment.

Consumers, if not asked in advance, will make their judgments known by requesting some doctors in the group more often than others, by preferring certain clinic locations, or by joining particular HMOs because the services provided are more suited to their needs than those offered in other HMOs or fee-for-service alternatives. Therefore, the involvement of the potential customer in determining strategy is fundamental to the process of developing marketing plans.

Logic Is Often Woefully Inadequate

Many times, individuals who are well intentioned become encumbered by such complications as company or clinic politics. For whatever reason, plans that fail to have appropriate logic are developed. This is a difficult problem to avoid and often even more difficult to solve. However, it should be noted that because an organization typically has numerous options, the logic of each marketing plan element should be closely scrutinized. Logic should be straightforward in order to minimize the lack of coherent or consistent plans for the organization and its markets.

Strategy Means Trade-Offs among Alternative Courses of Action

It is not possible to use all available strategies. By the same token, multiple strategies that the organization would like to achieve are often in conflict with one another. For example, a strategy for obtaining high growth through additional volume, based on an aggressive sales program, is in conflict with a strategy of high profitability. Simply stated, tremendous sales growth may be in conflict with maximum profitability. This is often one of the most difficult areas of strategy conflict. Yet, it is a reality of industry that dramatic growth costs money, which means that on a short-term basis, in order to achieve growth, profits may have to be diminished somewhat. The reason for this relates to the high cost of sales, promotion strategies, new investment intensity, such as capital required for new clinic locations, and related costs, such as staffing. For a clinic, this issue is a major obstacle because, often, individuals in the partnership do not want to sacrifice income to growth (especially if several of the partners are approaching retirement).

Market Share Is an Important Benchmark of Organizational Development

The value of market share as a performance indicator is often unrecognized in health care. Common standards of success are patient visits, patient days, gross revenue, or volume. While these are appropriate standards, considering these figures alone is deceptive. In a growing market, for example, the demand for home health care may be increasing. An organization is seeing more volume each quarter in this service area. The conclusion is that home health care is a successful service offering. Yet the hospital does not consider market share. With competitors in the market, the organization might experience increasing volume but at a lower rate of growth than its competitors. As the demand for home health care matures, the hospital may find itself with a small, unprofitable share of the market to serve. Without monitoring market share, a false sense of performance may exist.

Diversification Is More Difficult than One Would Expect

As health care businesses look at the problems confronting them in their primary business (such as the difficulties outlined in Chapter 1), it is often found that these hospitals, clinics, and related health care businesses spend a good deal of time exploring diversification opportunities. In fact, in the health care community, diversification as method of generating new revenue sources has become very popular. Although diversification is an important strategy which should not be overlooked, it can also be very risky.

An analysis of diversification attempts by the top 200 of the Fortune 500 corporations found that only a few businesses (18 percent) achieved profits in the first few years of diversification.[4] New ventures need, on the average, eight years before they reach profitability and approximately 12 years to reach cash flows similar to those of a mature business. Clearly, it would be dangerous to extrapolate this data directly to the health care environment. However, it is useful to know that the Fortune 500 companies from which this data was drawn are among the best-managed organizations

---

[4]Ralph Biggadike, ''The Risky Business of Diversification,'' *Harvard Business Review*, May/ June 1979, p. 103.

in the country, and often have greater knowledge than most health care organizations do in terms of diversification attempts.

Each Service or Business Needs a Competitive Advantage

Health care organizations need to develop market plans that will ultimately provide a competitive advantage in the marketplace. This advantage could be the best location, quickest response, best care, one-stop-service, or a variety of alternatives. A medical group often thinks it has a competitive advantage in being the "best doctors," for example, because all are board certified. Whereas this is important, the market may not recognize this advantage. In fact, the market may not recognize that the group has any advantage at all. Marketing plans try to seek a bona fide competitive advantage, from the market's perspective, which can be communicated and used to fix the clinic, hospital, or health care business in the mind of the consumer. For example, 7up's competitive advantage is no caffeine, Mayo Clinic has the competitive advantage of diagnostic excellence, and Hill Rom Hospital Furniture is known as a premium product. In all cases the competitive advantage is used to develop an enviable niche which sets one service apart from the others and creates marketplace awareness, interest, and ultimate utilization.

"Diversion and Dissuasion" Need to Be Utilized

Often an important strategy is to get the competition to think that you won't invest in a given opportunity or that the opportunity in which you have invested is so unimportant it doesn't warrant attention.[5] These strategies might also lead your competitor to believe that in direct competition, you will be able to crush them.

These tactics are common in business and are used to diminish the probability that a competitor will open across the street, develop a new service line, or compete for the same market segment.

For hospitals, the use of "diversion and dissuasion" tactics is often very difficult. Most hospitals have policies that allow the medical staff executive committee or general staff to approve new service offerings. Many times, physicians who participate in these discussions have staff appointments at two or three hospitals. As a result, information about a new program at General Hospital is often quickly available at Memorial Hospital, a situation which limits the capability to use these classical and necessary tactics.

As hospitals and physicians consider more joint ventures, problems of diversion and dissuasion are likely to become more important. As attempts are made to balance the need for "tactical surprise" versus traditional policy

---

[5]Henderson, *Henderson on Corporate Strategy*, p. 14.

versus physician vested interests versus hospital vested interests versus a competitive environment, hospitals and clinics will need to evaluate and develop ways to apropriately use these tactics.

Growth Is Often with Your Present Market

A common strategy for many organizations is to search for new markets, such as new physicians to bring on staff or more primary care physicians to enhance the clinic's referral base. Little time is spent, however, in increasing the loyalty of current existing users. As organizations develop their marketing plans, it is important to recognize that present buyers are as important as new users. Often increasing the loyalty (or usage rate) of existing buyers is less costly to achieve than attracting someone to the clinic who has never used the facility.

Is the Magnitude of Impact of the Marketing Plan Important within the Context of the Organization?

Excellent marketing plans are often developed for services that currently have or are destined to have only a minor impact on the hospital or clinic. Hospitals often develop small new programs and services which total less than 10 percent of the hospital operation. Yet, no marketing plans may be underway to enhance or modify services which constitute 90 percent of the business and are the backbone of the enterprise. Therefore, the strategic mind set must first concentrate on areas where the greatest impact can be made.

■ Summary

Before starting the marketing planning process, these elements, which constitute the strategic mind set, should be reviewed. If a reluctance to accept this mind set exists, it will be difficult to develop effective marketing plans.
    The strategic mind set consists of:

1. Services cannot remain static; change is inevitable.
2. There is often a better way and often the competitor will find it.
3. The marketplace has a decision-making role in helping to direct the future course of a business.
4. Logic is often woefully inadequate.
5. Strategy means trade-offs among alternative courses of action.
6. Market share is an important benchmark of organizational development.
7. Diversification is more difficult than one would expect.
8. Each service or business needs a competitive advantage.

9. Diversion and dissuasion need to be utilized.
10. Growth is often with your present market.
11. Is the magnitude of impact of the marketing plan important within the context of the organization?

The concepts within the strategic mind set involve the recognition that: (1) change is unavoidable—even with the best of products and services; (2) business tactics are applicable to the operation of health care organizations; and (3) the market upon which you depend (consumer, buyer, end user, patient, referring doctor) has a role in making decisions. Within the framework of this mind set the remainder of this book will address the development of a model for creating marketing plans in health care organizations.

Reference

Michael Porter. *Competitive Strategy*. New York: The Free Press, 1980.

CHAPTER 3

OUTLINING THE MARKETING PLANNING PROCESS

■ Relating the Market Plan to the Business Plan

Planning an organization's business activities is a complex process. Some of the many steps involved include goal-setting, identifying objectives, describing tasks, forecasting, setting quotas, monitoring performance, and budgeting. Types of planning activities include market planning, strategic planning, business planning, and long-range planning.

Each operating unit of the organization is responsible for producing its own distinct business plan *which incorporates the operational, financial, personnel and marketing needs of the specific unit*. These individual business plans, in turn, must fit into an overall operating plan—the organization's strategic plan. *The strategic business plan coordinates all of the organization's functional plans and is developed in light of the competitive environment.*

The business plan is an integral part of strategy formulation. As shown in Exhibit 3–1, the organization's first planning step is to develop a statement of mission and objectives. Following the mission and objective sequence is the important market plan. The market plan feeds the operations plan, which in turn feeds the personnel plan, which then feeds the financial plan. All of these items combine to make a *business plan*. Within each of these planning elements, there are goals, objectives, strategies, tasks, forecasts, quotas, budgets, and other appropriate items unique to each functional area. In marketing-oriented institutions, the market plan begins the planning

EXHIBIT 3–1
Organization Business Planning Process

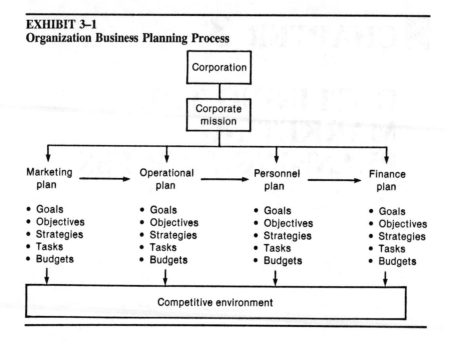

process and, through its external orientation, helps provide definition and direction for other functional areas.

In a multiunit corporate organization, each business should undertake this business planning activity. In a multispecialty clinic or a hospital, the planning activity should be done at the departmental level. Each service or program of the business should have its own marketing, financial, operations, and personnel plans as shown in Exhibit 3–2.

Combining the plans of each department within the hospital or clinic results in the overall strategic plan for the organization. For example, the rehabilitation department of a hospital may have as its mission, "to act as a feeder for other more profitable businesses within the organization." Surgery, on the other hand, may consider its objective to be, "providing enough cash and resources for profitability and development of additional hospital services." All of these activities, taken together, form the strategic plan, but before the strategic plan is put into action, the consistency of each business plan with the others must be insured.

A great deal of confusion exists regarding the relationship of planning to marketing. Arguments have been made that a corporate plan should be established before a marketing plan.[1] The concept advanced in this book is

[1] J. C. Higgins, *Strategic and Operational Systems*, (Englewood Cliffs, N.J.: Prentice-Hall, 1980). D. E. Hussey, *Corporate Planning*, (Elmsford, N.Y.: Pergamon Press, 1979).

EXHIBIT 3–2
The Organization Portfolio

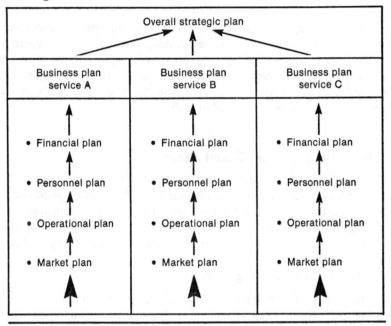

that planning is an integrative function in which interplay is constant between major management functions. For example, the mission is set within the context of marketplace forces, and the market plan is set within the context of mission and goals. Although this is an interactive process, the major premise of this book is that marketing plays a key first-step role in helping strategic planning determine which business to be in, and by providing a foundation for finance and other input areas in formulating these plans.

More confusion exists regarding planning in health care. Part of this relates to the way that planning was introduced into the health care environment. Typically, in many health care organizatons, planning began as the department which handled government regulatory affairs, such as health systems agencies or health planning councils. The first planner in most hospitals helped guide the organization through the regulatory process, but that person really did not participate in developing strategic direction for the organization.

In recent years, the role of the planner has evolved beyond regulatory activities and toward the development of long-range plans. Even now many hospital's long-range planning documents are often requested by health systems agencies. Many organizations, however, only develop plans because they are required by a local regulatory agency. Because clinics and other providers of medical care are largely unaffected by similar regulatory activities, the formal planning process has often not been part of their business operation.

Improvement in the development of the planning process has occurred. However, most organizations, if they develop plans, do not incorporate a market-based approach. The typical process is to begin with the wants and needs of people *in the hospital or clinic* and their view of the marketplace. The market-based approach starts with customer wants and needs and designs the program or service to address those needs.

■ Developing Market-Based Plans

In order to effectively accomplish marketing planning, it is necessary to have an understanding of what is meant by the term, "marketing philosophy." There is much information about this concept and its implementation.

The marketing philosophy is quite simple, but despite its simplicity, most organizations have never been successful in understanding or implementing the concept.

Basically, the marketing concept is:

1. The process of listening to consumers and the marketplace.
2. The philosophy of organizing to *satisfy needs* of a group or groups of consumers.
3. The satisfaction of these needs in a profitable fashion.

The essence of marketing is best highlighted by eight points.

EXHIBIT 3-3
The Essence of Marketing

Marketing is:

1. A philosophy of consumer orientation.
2. Managing by objectives.
3. A system of commercial intelligence.
4. A road to dynamic business strategy.
5. A process of business planning.
6. An emphasis on innovation.
7. A means of performance evaluation.
8. A focus for future opportunities.

The manager must understand that planning starts with marketing. Marketing plans are an integrative process of listening to the marketplace and developing strategies and objectives that both meet the guidelines of the organization and are realistic within the context of financial and operating parameters. We shall now turn to an overview of the marketing planning process, which will be used throughout the remainder of this manual.

■ An Overview of the Process

A marketing plan starts by analyzing the market. Most health care organizations think of their internal needs first and the marketplace second. This is a nonmarket-based approach. A market-oriented manager, however, begins with external needs and uses them to focus internal actions. This is a market-based approach. Exhibit 3–4 presents a nonmarket-based and a market-based planning approach. As can be seen, the two approaches vary in just a few instances. Yet the dramatic difference between these two planning approaches may best be seen only by example.

In a nonmarket-based model, the board of directors, as physician shareholders in the group, establish the goals and objectives for the organization. Then, typically, these individuals set the goals for the coming planning period. At Brighton Hospital, for example, the mission is to provide high quality care to residents of the immediate community. On the planning committee are two physicians who have had a long-standing relationship with the hospital and are respected by their peers. Both physicians have served as former chiefs of the medical staff. These physicians believe there is a need to establish a basic rehabilitation program in their area. Discussions at medical meetings and articles in popular trade journals suggest that such programs are increasingly common. Based on the political persuasion of these physicians, a decision is made to allocate resources and space to a full clinic. The program is set to open in 60 days. One week before the opening, concern starts to rise. The public relations department is instructed to build demand through immediate media coverage. Six months after taking the service to market, demand does not meet projections.

How would this scenario change under a market-based approach? The organization members still set their mission. Yet the fulfillment of this mission is accomplished with direction from the market. Needs are assessed at the start. What are the opportunities for a rehabilitation program? Potential referral physicians see little need or advantage for this program, yet report referral needs on sports medicine. Does a sports medicine program fit within the mission? Yes. The design of the program is laid out. Before full-scale implementation is achieved, the program is tested. A sample of physicians review the proposed program. Hours, costs, and planned patient procedures are described. What is the market's reaction? If this program is not what the referral physicians had in mind, the proposal may have to be reformulated before going to market. If acceptable, the task becomes one of *informing* the market that the *service* which they desired is now available in the configuration they suggested—at an acceptable *price,* with the desired range of services established in an accessible manner.

EXHIBIT 3–4
Internal Planning versus Marketing Planning

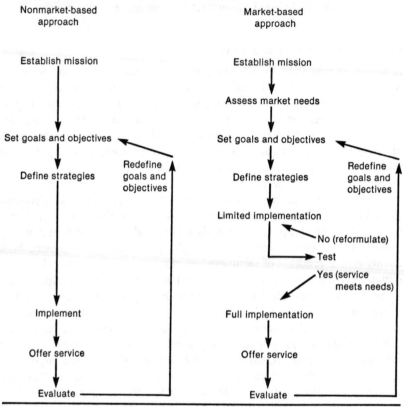

A market-based approach is not "right" and the nonmarket approach "wrong." Yet as financial resources became more restricted, the cost of mistakes (in terms of programs not meeting expectations) is more serious for the organization. A market-based approach helps improve the odds for success. It should be easier to listen to the market and provide the necessary programs than to attempt to divine what buyers might need. There are six basic steps, then, in establishing effective marketing plans.

The Marketing Planning Sequence

1. Setting the mission.
2. An internal/external analysis.
3. Determining the strategy action match and marketing objectives.
4. Developing action strategies.
5. Integrating the plan and making revisions.

6. Providing appropriate control procedures, feedback, and integration of all plans into a unified effort.

These six steps form the basis of this book. At each step, there are three types of activities which are necessary for success. First, the process of doing the necessary staff work to support decision making; second, the process of actually making decisions; and third, integration with other business units or services to enhance coordination between the functional units, such as operations and finance. As each step and its component parts is diagramed, it will be done in relation to these three activities. Therefore, the flow chart of the marketing planning process ingredients will be shown in the following sequence. (See Exhibit 3–5.)

EXHIBIT 3–5
The Planning Process Ingredients

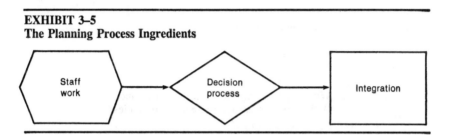

Staff work represents the collection of detail and data needed in the decision-making process. Here, marketing plans differ substantially from other planning approaches. In addition to internal data, the market plan model depends heavily on attitudes, opinions, and the environment of those outside the organization. It does not rely solely on management's point of view. Thus, staff work includes the gathering of data on both internal and external markets.

This marketing orientation also requires that health care professionals be willing to accept the fact that the marketplace should have an impact on decision making. For example, growth of a clinic could be predicated on new office hours based on expressed consumer need, or a clinic's contract with an HMO could be based on consumer demand.

It is within the middle category, the decision process, that the actual steps of a marketing plan will be charted. As the organization assesses the external market data, decisions must be made on how to react to external conditions in light of the hospital's or clinic's internal capabilities.

The last category, the integration process, includes those activities which involve the integration of marketing plans with finance, personnel, operations, and resource allocation. Also included here are the development of the organization's entire product or service portfolio and the sharing and coordination of plans with the other services within the health care organization.

Many organizations talk about planning without really understanding what it means. Some have a reasonably good system for determining and controlling expenses and then mistakenly believe that this is an annual planning or market planning process. Other companies confuse budgeting with planning. While budgeting and forecasting are important in the development of market plans, they are not the sole ingredients for a market plan which, when completed, will contain answers to the questions in Exhibit 3–6.

EXHIBIT 3–6
The Market Planning Questions

Where is the market?
 1. Needs and demands.
Where are you now?
 2. As an institution?
 3. As a department?
 4. As an individual?
 5. With respect to the environment and competition?
 6. With respect to capabilities and opportunities?
Where do you want to go?
 7. Assumptions/potentials.
 8. Objectives and goals.
How do you want to get there?
 9. Policies and procedures/levels of initiative.
10. Strategies and programs.
When do you want to arrive?
11. Priorities and schedules.
Who is responsible?
12. Organization and delegation.
How much will it cost?
13. Budgets and resource allocations?
How will we know if we did it?
14. Feedback and review sessions.
15. Continuous monitoring.

The marketing planning approach involves the six steps listed previously, the necessary staff work, management decisions, and functional integration. The marketing model which incorporates these elements is shown in Exhibit 3–7.

It would be possible to develop a plan by just using the middle column of the diagram (Exhibit 3–7) without regard for either staff work or functional integration. In fact, many health care organizations currently operate

EXHIBIT 3–7
The Marketing Planning Model

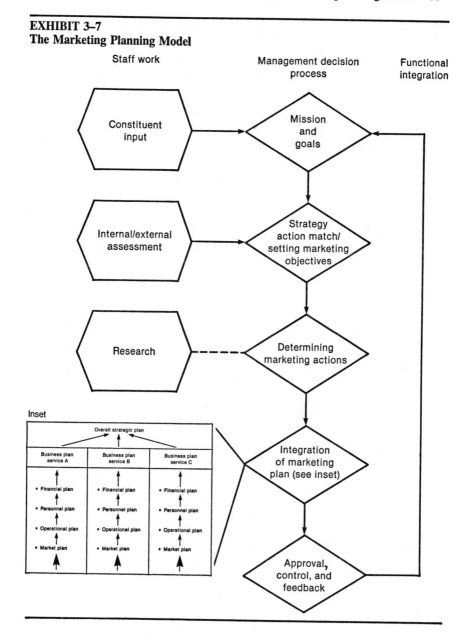

this way. Missions are set, some marketing goals are specified, and strategies implemented. However, that approach is not a market plan.

To establish an effective marketing plan, it is necessary to understand the first premise of marketing. Marketing is the process of *understanding* customer wants and needs, *listening* to those wants and needs, and then, to whatever extent possible, *designing* appropriate programs and services to meet those wants and needs in a timely, cost-effective, competitive fashion. *It is the process of molding the organization to the market, rather than convincing the market that the organization (for example, a clinic) provides what they need.*

This is the necessary foundation for generating a market plan. In addition, a successful market plan must be developed in relationship to other pressures and functions within the organization. The need for integration is critical to successful implementation. (See Exhibit 3–5.)

The requirements for the successful development of a market plan are simple. These are shown in Exhibit 3–8.

EXHIBIT 3–8
The Requirements for Successful Marketing Plan Development

1. Top management must be committed to the process.
2. The CEO is the chief strategist.
3. Marketing plans must be a way of life, not something that occurs during a certain time within the business year.
4. The approach must be balanced and integrative.
5. There must be detailed goals.
6. There must be an action plan.
7. The action plan must be results oriented.

CHAPTER 4

ESTABLISHING THE MISSION—STEP 1

Step 1: Establishing the Mission

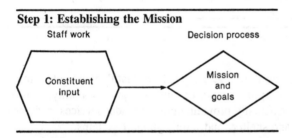

Determining the mission and setting goals are functions of the organization's governing authority. The board may spend a great deal of direct time involved in discussing these topics. It is the responsibility of the staff, however, to develop appropriate information upon which the governing authority can act. In this chapter the mission and goal-setting process is described. While the nature of staff work in supporting mission and goal-setting *often* varies by organization, the general scope of this activity is discussed.

■ Defining the Mission

The development of a statement of business mission (or purpose) has become popular. Every group seems to have one. Samples of varying mission statements are shown in Exhibit 4–1.

These organizations are often addressing the question, What business are we in? It is very easy for hospitals, clinics, and nursing homes to be

EXHIBIT 4−1
Sample Corporate Mission Statements

> The mission of United Hospitals, Inc., is to provide the best possible health care services to meet the health and illness needs of persons in the community we serve and to exercise corporate leadership in organizing and supporting health care resources through a diversified multiunit system organization.
>
> Hospital Corporation of America is the world's leading hospital management company. The company was founded with the fundamental belief that private enterprise can deliver quality health care at a reasonable cost using private capital, paying all property and income taxes, and providing superior facilities and equipment. In pursuing this policy, the company is consciously working to contain the rising cost of health care and to provide its shareholders a fair return on their investment.
>
> The mission of Fairview Community Hospitals is to provide high quality health-related services in a spirit of Christian concern to meet the personal needs and improve the health status of the people and communities we serve.

myopic in their thinking. They believe that they are solely in the business of operating a hospital, clinic, or nursing home. In reality, most of these organizations are actually providing much broader services, such as health education, care and shelter, and family support systems.

While some organizations may have become rather broad based in their approach to business, their statements of mission are often still very narrow. Along with a limited clinic or hospital mission comes myopic thinking regarding future options for the organization. As a business matures, a narrow mission statement can restrict the examination of potential growth opportunities. For example, banks can't afford to be in "banking." They must be in "financial services" in order to grow in their complex marketplace.

For growth to occur, it will often be necessary for hospitals to begin to think outside the traditional definition of a hospital. It is important for the health care organization to define as appropriately as possible, in a rather broad context, its general mission. For example, two hospitals may state that they are in health care. One hospital might be rather narrow and suggest that it is in the mission of health care in an urban setting, operating within a religious framework. The second hospital has a broader mission statement specifying its business as providing health care services.

When the first hospital looks at opportunities, it considers traditional programs which are geographically constrained. The second organization looks toward providing a range of health care services where needed. This organization has decided to use some space on the hospital grounds to install an indoor running track. After 5 P.M., the pool used during the day for physical therapy will be available for open swimming. The hospital also hopes to offer a health and exercise program with hospital nutritionists providing appropriate assistance in dietary planning. There is discussion at the hospital to contract with corporations, as well as with police and fire departments, to join the program. For an additional charge, a physical exam would be included. This hospital also plans to provide support to four primary care physicians in opening a satellite office in a community where residents expressed a desire for greater accessibility to routine medical care.

In order to arrive at a mission statement for a health care organization, it is valuable to have input from the various constituencies of the hospital or clinic. A difficulty in developing market-based plans in health care is the number of constituencies whose opinions must be assessed. Examples of these many groups are shown in Exhibit 4–2.

EXHIBIT 4–2
Potential Constituents Who Influence the Mission

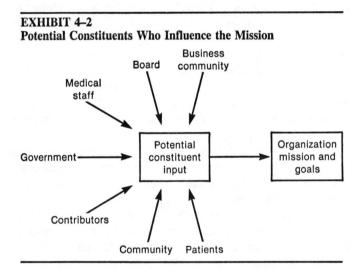

Development of a corporate mission statement will address the question, What business are we in? To answer, input is needed from the critical constituencies. Often these views will differ in direction or focus. To aid in integrating this diverse input, each constituency group should be asked to address common issues. Exhibit 4–3 outlines these areas in the form of seven questions.

These questions thoroughly examine the historical purpose of the organization. They also analyze the corporate value structure. However, specifications of mission must consider existing relationships with various groups. For example, the organization might be strongly associated with the Catholic community of a particular diocese within a city. This relationship may be reflected in the mission.

EXHIBIT 4-3
Required Constituent Inputs

1. What is the history and heritage of the organization?
2. What are the historical relationships of the organization?
3. What prior relationships, formal and informal, have been arranged, developed, and nurtured that have an impact on the organization?
4. What is the corporate value structure of management, the board of trustees and the constituencies of the organization?
5. What is the value structure of the people that this organization serves?
6. What is the probable future of the external environment?
7. What corporate resources are likely to be available in the foreseeable future to support the corporate mission?

It is important for all concerned to recognize how different missions could lead to different implementation strategies. For example, assume that a hospital establishes a family practice clinic combined with an after-hours emergency service. This facility is located in an urban area 10 miles from the sponsoring hospital. Depending on the established mission of the family practice clinic, and particularly the emergency care service, it would be possible to have a variety of outcomes.

One alternative mission of the emergency care component could be to *act as a funnel of new patients* to the family practice clinic. The purpose would be to attract patients for ongoing care in the ambulatory setting. This mission would call for a set of aggressive marketing strategies designed to attract virtually all patients in the area, whether they had a physician or not. An alternative mission of the facility might be to support physician practices in the area. A specific goal would be to *build the practice* of the private clinic, not through aggressive marketing to patients, but rather through the emergency care center communicating its support function to all area physicians. Again, the decision would depend on the mission selected.

■ Specifying the Goals

Once the health care organization has decided on a business mission, it is possible to establish its goals. In most cases, these goals should be few in number. Management should keep in mind that the more goals it establishes, the greater the tendency to limit available strategic alternatives. Over-specification can result in these goals serving as constraints to management action.

Normally, goal statements address three major areas: *Profitability* is usually stated in financial terms, such as return on investment. The *desired growth* for the clinic is also included, as well as *potential new areas of business*. An example of some selected goal statements is shown in Exhibit 4-4.

EXHIBIT 4-4
Alternative Goal Statements

Provide complete range of health care services to the community at large.

Maintain 16 percent return on investment by investing in health-related businesses.

Expand to become the largest health care provider in the region in order to maintain a mission of healing.

Prepare organization for sellout.

Become a multispecialty clinic with a regional reputation for oncology.

Presidents and senior advisors should realize, however, that the corporate mission and goal statement is not the place for detailed operating objectives. In order to maximize flexibility and allow the process of strategy development to take place, the mission statement should provide the broadest possible context for overall organization direction. For example, a clinic which states as its mission, "to meet the health needs of the community through health-related services," has provided direction and limitations. Investment strategies might call for development of a prosthetics supply house. Yet investment of clinic money in a condominium development, while offering a higher rate of return for the group, would not be appropriate. In summary, corporate goals should help set the tone, pace and general direction of the health care organization.

In order to take this first step in developing a market plan, an integra tion activity must occucr. Input from finance, operations, marketing, and other interest groups is required at the start in order to have successful implementation at the end. This decision regarding the mission statement cannot be made in a vacuum without market, financial, or operational data.

■ Mission Statement Checklist

The purpose of this chapter was to develop a mission statement for the organization. It is this statement which will provide the parameters in which marketing plans can be developed. Listed below are several checklist questions to review regarding specifications of the organization mission. Again, recalling the sequence of the market-based approach, needs are not assessed until the mission is specified. This statement serves to provide direction for the range of needs which might be considered relevant for future actions.

1. Does the mission of your organization reflect a broad enough orientation and provide flexibility to make changes as required?
2. Did all important constituencies have an opportunity to provide input or comment on the mission?

3. Did your organization work through possible alternative operating scenarios to see how the mission might be applied? Specifically, did the mission provide guidance as to what types of scenarios are acceptable and not acceptable?
4. Does the mission provide a set of goals that are specific enough to give guidance to the organization, yet broad enough to provide flexibility?

▨ CHAPTER 5

CONDUCTING THE INTERNAL/EXTERNAL ASSESSMENT—STEP 2

A competitive marketing plan is based upon clearly defined marketing objectives. Establishing marketing objectives (short-range, result-oriented) is based on two perspectives. The first perspective is the purpose and mission of the organization determined in step 1. The second perspective is the detailed internal/external analysis which includes evaluation of competitors, internal analysis, market research, segmentation, and service evaluation. Accomplishing step 2 in the most appropriate fashion requires keeping corporate purposes and missions in mind, but setting the actual goals in relation to the marketplace. In other words, design your business around the consumer. This is a strategy used by successful companies and is "one of the best-kept secrets in American business" according to Peters and Waterman in a book entitled, *In Search of Excellence.*[1]

Step 2 consists of the environmental analysis and the strategy action match. Marketing objectives are subsequently determined. The detail required in this step and its importance to the overall planning process cannot be overestimated. In this chapter specific attention is paid to the internal/external analysis. The four components of this phase of step 2 are shown on page 44. Discussion of the strategy action match and objective setting is presented in Chapter 6.

Establishing marketing objectives follows naturally from an understanding of the general tone of the corporate mission statement and objectives. Marketing objectives represent specific targets which the organization

---

[1]Thomas Peters and Robert Waterman, *In Search of Excellence*, (New York: Harper & Row, 1982), p. 157.

Step Two: Conducting the Internal/External Assessment

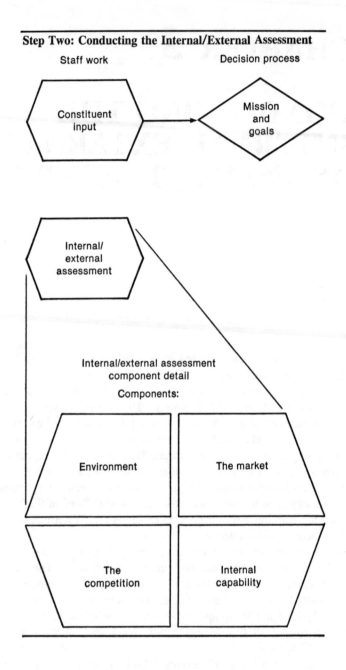

will move toward over the next one to two years. Setting those objectives depends on information from the internal/external analysis. This analysis, although time-consuming, is a critical phase in the development of market plans. It may uncover numerous opportunities for the organization to consider. Management must be careful to concentrate resources on objectives and opportunities that: (1) fit the mission, and (2) provide the greatest reward.

■ Conducting the Internal/External Analysis

In a sense, the internal/external analysis is the foundation of the marketing plan—the set of assumptions on which the entire plan is built. If the analysis is inadequate, incomplete, or untruthful, the entire plan will suffer. Most organizations starting on a market plan for the first time assume they know all of the necessary information, have adequate data, and need not spend much time on this phase of step 2. However, by going through this process, an organization usually uncovers new opportunities and ideas, along with a better analysis of organizational weaknesses.

To many who have never undertaken an internal/external analysis, the process may seem elementary. The attitude of some managers is that by virtue of having been involved in a particular hospital or clinic for years, they know where they are and where they ought to go. They mistakenly think that the internal/external analysis is unnecessary. Although this process often requires a month or more of staff time and some intraorganizational stress, the thought-provoking inquiry produces valuable marketing insights.

The internal/external analysis is the foundation of the market approach —that is, to listen, to inquire, to study, and to ask questions. Therefore, an examination of those questions which are most important in the establishment and process of conducting the internal/external analysis will be reviewed. This analysis and situation review encompasses several major areas:

The environment.
The market and its needs.
The competition.
Internal capabilities.
The marketing function and programs.

Many organizations are able to conduct the analysis internally. In this instance, the internal/external analysis is typically the responsibility of one individual who, through the support of others on the staff, will gather the necessary information to answer each of the detailed questions. It is possible to conduct an internal/external analysis for an entire organization. However, as the organization grows larger, it becomes more meaningful for the analysis to be done on a departmental or service-by-service basis. In other words, a small clinic of three to five practitioners could effectively conduct a single internal/external analysis. On the other hand, a 400-bed hospital would get the most value out of conducting an analysis on a department-by-department basis. Large, complex organizations often find it necessary to use outside consultants to conduct the internal/external analysis. However, the questions typically asked within an analysis are similar, whether conducted by an outside consultant or internal staff. Often an outside facilitator can ensure that critical questions are answered, regardless of political sensitivity.

The purpose of the analysis is to uncover marketing opportunities and threats. The internal strengths and weaknesses of the firm are examined, as are the opportunities present externally. Several questions must be addressed within each component of the analysis. These areas are reviewed in the following pages.

■ The Environment

The first component of the internal/external analysis is an understanding of the macroenvironment. Information from a variety of sources is gathered in order to make judgments regarding opportunities, threats, and future business outlook. This information will eventually be matched to an assessment of the organization's capabilities and weaknesses.

Exhibit 5–1 contains the "External Marketplace Assessment" form. This chart is a quick and useful first step. This assessment should be conducted on a program or service basis. The object of this exercise is to ensure that the hospital or clinic has considered the major factors which could have an impact on the future of the program. Included within this assessment are several global questions pertaining to the marketplace. How large is the market and what is its growth potential? Competitive factors must also be addressed, along with factors that might change the nature of competition, such as technology, financial concerns of investment, and reimbursement.

For each program, the manager must provide some indication of market attractiveness. A judgment is asked for in terms of present conditions and conditions over the next three years. These judgments are provided on the scale of "high–medium–low." An essential first step for any organization is to define the scale points. Because operating scale varies for an acute care hospital, a tertiary facility, or 10-person, multispecialty clinic; the scale values must be determined by each organization. For example, a 3 percent predicted growth in the market may not be attractive to a clinic operating at near capacity, but this level might be highly attractive to a group needing revenue flow.

Because this review is suggested as a first-cut evaluation of multiple programs, data should be gathered from existing sources. And since the regulatory environment affects the health care industry to a greater extent than many other industries, this environmental factor must always be monitored. Because regulations often vary by program, several specific regulatory questions should be posed for the major service areas.

EXHIBIT 5–1
External Marketplace Assessment

| Service_____ | Market Attractiveness | | | | | |
| | Current | | | 3 Yrs. Forward | | |
	High	Med	Low	High	Med	Low
Size of market						
Growth rate						
Stage of life cycle						
Price stability						
Distribution requirements						
Service requirements						
Level of technology						
Potential for functional substitution						
Captive patients						
Customer concentration						
Degree of competition						
Attitude—passive? aggressive?						
Number of competitors						
Strength of leader						
Service profitability						
Leverage potential, e.g., economies of scale						
Service intensity						
Service capacity utilization						
Social attitudes/trends						
Reimbursement climate						
Regulatory exposure/vulnerability						
Overall market attractiveness						

Conclusion:

1. What kinds of external controls affect your organization:
    Local?

    State?

    Federal?

    Self-regulatory?

2. What are the trends in recent regulatory rulings?

EXHIBIT 5–2
Identification of Major Markets and Needs

Part I—Identify markets. A market or market segment consists of a group of people who have common demographic, specialty, or social characteristics that represent a size large enough for the organization to concentrate resources around.

Potential Markets	Importance of Market (check one column for current and future)						Current Attitude Toward You (circle one number)				
	Current			Future			Very Favorable				Very Unfavorable
	High	Med	Low	High	Med	Low	1	2	3	4	5
Gen. medicine M.D.'s							1	2	3	4	5
Surgeons							1	2	3	4	5
OB/gyn							1	2	3	4	5
Peds							1	2	3	4	5
Other M.D.'s							1	2	3	4	5
Inpatients (by specialty)							1	2	3	4	5
Outpatients							1	2	3	4	5
Community at large							1	2	3	4	5
Donors							1	2	3	4	5
Board of directors							1	2	3	4	5
Insurance companies							1	2	3	4	5
Regulators							1	2	3	4	5
Business/ industry (specify)							1	2	3	4	5
Have no doctor market							1	2	3	4	5
							1	2	3	4	5
HMO patients							1	2	3	4	5
Over-65 market							1	2	3	4	5
Nonuser market							1	2	3	4	5
Females							1	2	3	4	5
Males							1	2	3	4	5
Others_____							1	2	3	4	5
_____							1	2	3	4	5
_____							1	2	3	4	5
_____											

State and national professional associations, discussions with congressional staff members, and planning agency documents all should be used in this assessment. This procedure should be conducted at least yearly for each existing program within the facility.

EXHIBIT 5–2 *(concluded)*

Part II—Based on the mix of actual and potential markets listed in Part I, indicate the size and future potential.

Key Market Segments from Part I	Size Today	Future Size— Three Years	Your Current Market Share
25 thru 34-year-old males - athletics	9% of metro area	14%	32% of medical care needs in sports medicine programs

Part III—Based on completion of Parts I and II, indicate the needs major market segments are likely to exhibit.

Key Market Segments	Needs
25 thru 34 - year-old males in sports medicine program	Greater emphasis on strength training, cardiovascular fitness

■ The Market and Its Needs

The role of any market plan is to determine the major markets and their respective needs. This is the second component of the internal/external assessment. Exhibit 5–2 provides a quick check analysis of markets, similar to the external form just presented. Completing this analysis helps identify the major markets and appropriate segments.

As shown in Exhibit 5–2, the identified markets are both internal and external. Some organizations which have established foundations supporting the group's medical research activities may consider donors of high current importance. A second group may consider this segment to be of high future importance, as their clinic or hospital moves into research activities. For a religious hospital, the board of directors, which may have strong church input, might be of high current and future importance.

The list of markets shown in Exhibit 5–2 is in no way exhaustive. Some hospitals might prefer to identify their markets by race or geographic location in the city. The purpose of this identification sheet is to encourage the management team to explicitly state its relevant markets and the existing attitude (or support) of those markets to the service offered.

The second and third parts of the market identification form require a deeper consideration of the organization's key segments. Forecasting the future size of market segments is essential. A common problem for many organizations is the identification of a key segment and the realization of future decline. The third part of Exhibit 5–2 forces a marketing perspective to the key segments. Members of the organization must consider what the *likely* needs are for these groups. Lack of knowledge of future needs will highlight an information gap for market research.

Data to complete the form can be obtained from several sources. Opinions of staff members are valuable. In addition, it is useful to examine billing files, medical records and physician index reports. Often this analysis results in learning that the *actual* markets served by the group differ from those perceived by its members.

In the provision of health care, little can be done without the physician, the primary deliverer of the service. Because of the significance of this market to a hospital trying to attract (or retain) medical staff loyalty, or to a group practice needing productive members, a separate review is necessary. Exhibit 5–3 is a suggested format for analysis of physician staff activity.

Data on several dimensions are necessary to work through this format. Specifically:

Age of physician.

Specialty.

Location of practice.

Practice type (for hospital).

Years on staff.

Utilization by number of patient days.

Dollars billed.

Surgeries.

Share of total hospital procedures.

For the hospital, a staff review provides a perspective on who are the major producers. Moreover, it identifies individuals whose practices are developing or who are beginning to shift their case loads to another facility. Typically, in any organization, a small group of physicians accounts for a disproportionate share of the volume. This group must be identified, and its loyalty maintained. Likewise, the age of this group might necessitate recruiting needs of varying levels of immediacy.

Recognizing or identifying the organization's markets is the basic step to developing effective marketing strategies. Listed below are several questions which management should consider in its market determination. These issues are far more detailed than those addressed in the market identification form.

EXHIBIT 5 – 3
Analysis of Physician Staff

List Staff	Age	Specialty	$ Billed 19___	Activity 19___	19___	Percent Change
_____	_____	_____	_____	_____	_____	_____
_____	_____	_____	_____	_____	_____	_____
_____	_____	_____	_____	_____	_____	_____
_____	_____	_____	_____	_____	_____	_____

Identify those that do 80 percent of activity (or billed revenue) in facility for further analysis.

Name	Age	Specialty	$ Billed 19___	Activity 19___	19___	Percent Change
_____	_____	_____	_____	_____	_____	_____
_____	_____	_____	_____	_____	_____	_____
_____	_____	_____	_____	_____	_____	_____
_____	_____	_____	_____	_____	_____	_____

Specifically, overall changes must be considered which are beyond the control of the organization.

1. What are the main developments with respect to demography, economy, technology, government, and culture that will affect the organization's situation?

In answering question 1, many organizations have found that the demographics of their communities have necessitated changes in the specialty composition of their group, or the program offered by their hospital.

2. Who are the organization's major markets and publics?
3. How large is the service area covered by your market?
4. What are the major segments in each market?
5. What are the present and expected future size profit and characteristics of each market or market segment?
6. What is the expected rate of growth of each segment?

The preceding questions require an inspection of who the organization serves. One tertiary facility determined the area from which its patients originated (question 3). Although the hospital always believed it drew its patients from three states, answering this question results in a different perspective. Seventy-five percent of the patients were found to come from seven counties around the hospital (all in the same state). This finding led to a different focus for promotion efforts, as well as the physician outreach program.

7. How fast and far have markets expanded?
8. Where do your patients come from geographically?

The remaining 11 questions pertain to *why* your market(s) buy or use your service.

9. What are the benefits which customers in different segments derive from the product: economics, better performance, displaceable cost, etc.?
10. What are the reasons for buying the product in different segments: product features, awareness, price, advertising, promotion, packaging, display, sales assistance, etc.?
11. What is the market standing with established customers in each segment: market share, pattern of repeat business, expansion of customers' product use, etc.?
12. What are the requirements for success in each market?
13. What are the customer attitudes in different segments: brand awareness, brand image (mapping), etc.?
14. What is the overall reputation of the product in each segment?
15. What are the reasons which reinforce the customer's faith in the company and product?
16. What are the reasons which force customers to turn elsewhere for help in using the product?

17. What is the life cycle status of the product?
18. What product research and improvements are planned?
19. Are there deficiencies in servicing or assisting customers in using the product?

For example, what are the benefits for which people use your clinic (question 9)? Is it technical skill or accessibility? If accessibility, how might your competition eliminate this advantage? Consider the impact of question 12—requirements for market success. If your market is after-hours care patients, what is required? Physician coverage may mean a new medical recruitment effort. A safe environment for the clinic is a necessity for night care. Where is the facility located?

It may not be possible to answer all questions because of personnel constraints or, more often, lack of knowledge. The value of this process is to identify where the organization needs to gather more data before specifying marketing action strategies.

■ The Competitive Environment

A third component of the internal/external analysis is an examination of existing and future competition. It is essential to realize that having a good product may not be enough if your competitors also have one. A thorough evaluation of competitor's strengths and weaknesses can help lead to a design for products and services which most competitively positions the clinic or hospital. It is important to develop an understanding not only of competitors' strengths and weaknesses, but also of their organizational capabilities and likely future thrusts. Once a thorough situation analysis is completed, reasonable objectives can be specified for action in addressing these areas.

A detailed analysis of competitors should be undertaken from an external view. As a first step, key issues to be addressed are who the competitors are, which competitors are likely to emerge, and where competitors are most vulnerable. A detailed competitor profile analysis is provided in Exhibit 5–4.

A complete fact sheet should be compiled on each major competitor. Unlike the profile form which was based on internal personnel's opinions, this competitive analysis should be based on as much objective external data available. Several sources may be helpful in completing this review, such as:

PSRO.

HSA—for C.O.N.s, market share.

American Hospital Association.

Health-related professional associations.

American Medical Association.

Other planning agencies.

Regional transit authority.

Chamber of Commerce.

Commercial research firms (such as Dun & Bradstreet).

EXHIBIT 5−4
Competitor Profile Form

Part I—Develop a competitor profile sheet on each relevant competitor.

A. Overview.
    Name of competitor:
    Size/volume: *19__   19__   19__   19__*

B. Nature of organization/operation (size, M.D. mix, type of org.).

C. Competitive strength.

D. Competitive weakness.

E. Likely key competitive moves.

F. Likely key long-range strategy.

Part II—Obtain market-share data on yourself and your competitors.

Market share is important because it tells how you are doing in relation to the competition.

	Share				
Competitor	*19__*	*19__*	*Percent Change*	*19__*	*Percent Change*
1.					
2.					
3.					
4.					
5.					
6.					

Bureau of the Census.
Drug/pharmaceutical companies.
Business/industrial organizations.
City and county directories.
Registration/licensure agencies.
Other government agencies/publications.

The first part of the competitor profile form is overview information. Several questions are detailed in the following pages to help focus on the necessary information. An important information need is the market share data for yourself and major competitors. Often, planning data can provide the necessary share data. Ignoring the organization's market share relative to the competition can have serious consequences.

Most groups evaluate their own absolute performance by patient days, gross revenue, or patient visits. This approach ignores the relative issue. A clinic's absolute number of patient visits could be growing in family practice, but its growth could be at a lower rate than the competition. Thus, the group is not attracting its proportion (or share) of new family practice business. Over time, the group may find itself having little impact in the market.

A second component to assessing competitive position is a relative assessment, done on several dimensions listed in Exhibit 5–5.

The objective of this evaluation is to provide an internal perspective on the organization's relative competitive position. Several key personnel should complete the form independently. For an organization to begin to develop plans and allocate resources to actions, some similarity of views on the external competition is important. Otherwise, conflict often occurs as different members perceive more or less concern from other groups or hospitals. The personal biases in completing this form are its strengths and weaknesses. Varying views on competitive position must be resolved early in the planning process.

The second part of the relative competitor assessment form requires a profile of "how competitive" another organization is and the basis for this competition.

On the following pages, several questions are raised to provide direction in addressing the competitive intensity issue and focusing on the basis of competition. It is important to overcome an organization's tendency to be myopic with regard to competition. Any clinic's competitive environment is very dynamic. As outlined in the first chapter, proprietary systems might move into a market area and dramatically change the nature of competition. If you compete in the same industry as a Humana, for example, recognition of its potential competitive threat is critical. What can your organization do to discourage entry into your market by a potential competitor? Consider then the following questions:

1. How many competitors are in your industry?
   How do you define your competitors?
   Has the number increased or decreased in the last four years?
2. What is your position in the market (size and strength) relative to competitors?
3. Who are the organization's major competitors?
4. What trends can be foreseen in competition?
5. Are there other companies that might be enticed to serve your customers or markets? This should include conglomerates or diversified companies that might be attracted by the growth, size or profitability of your markets. Choose the most likely new entries and consider what you know about them and their strategies.

EXHIBIT 5-5
The Relative Competitor Assessment Form
What's your profile?

Determine how you would rate each category in relation to your competition.

Competitor (specify): _____	Much Worse	Somewhat Worse		About the Same			Somewhat Better		Much Better
	−4	−3	−2	−1	0	+1	+2	+3	+4
1. Medical care									
A. Emergency									
B. Surgery									
C. Gen. medical									
D. Special care									
2. Nursing care									
3. Housekeeping (hospital)									
4. Food service (hospital)									
5. Staff morale									
6. Facility: Capacity/attractiveness									
7. Public relations									
8. Reputation									
9. Image (overall)									
10. Management									
11. Lab services									
13. Convenience									
14. Staff education									
15. Equipment: Capability/technology									
16. Range of services									
17. Marketing plan									
18. Ad/promo budget									

Competitive Assessment: For each competitor that you listed on the previous page, indicate the level of competitive intensity, your share of the market, and the basis for competition.

	Market Share	Level of Competitive Intensity						Basis for Competition			
		Very Intense		Not Competitive at All			Product	Price	Promotion	Distribution
1.	_____	1	2	3	4	5	_____	_____	_____	_____
2.	_____	1	2	3	4	5	_____	_____	_____	_____
3.	_____	1	2	3	4	5	_____	_____	_____	_____
4.	_____	1	2	3	4	5	_____	_____	_____	_____
5.	_____	1	2	3	4	5	_____	_____	_____	_____
6.	_____	1	2	3	4	5	_____	_____	_____	_____
7.	_____	1	2	3	4	5	_____	_____	_____	_____
8.	_____	1	2	3	4	5	_____	_____	_____	_____

Competitor

Conclusion: _____

58

6. What about companies on the periphery—those which serve the same customers with different but related products. This might include other pieces of equipment related to yours or equipment that would be included in a broader definition of the market. It is impossible to list all related items, but those of closest proximity should be included.

A major difficulty in the health care industry is the impact of technology. New technological development can mean the appearance of a new threat or the elimination of a hospital's competitive advantage. Two additional questions to focus thinking on this factor are:

7. List other products or services that provide the same or similar function. Record the percentage of total market sales for each substitute product.
8. Anticipate product innovations which could replace or reduce the sales of your products. When do you think these products will be commercially feasible? (Note: Information about potentially competitive products can be found by searching the records of U.S. Patent Office or foreign patent offices.)

Existing competition must always be considered. Of particular concern is the basis for competition. Is it on the service mix? Does the other group offer a broader range of specialties? Is it price competition, whereby the teaching hospital may be at a disadvantage to the Preferred Provider Organizations? It is important to understand the competitive thrust of others and their potential impact on your market share.

9. What are the choices afforded patients?
     In services?
     In payment?
10. Is competition based on a price or nonprice basis?
11. How do competitors (segment/price) advertise?

Finally, the organization's sensitivity to geographic susceptibility should always be maintained, and diversification strategies of those familiar with the industry should always be monitored. Think about:

12. Competitors in other geographic regions or other segments who do not currently compete in your markets or segments, but may decide to.
13. Customers served by our industry. Note those who may want to move backwards, and consider the reasons why such a move may make sense.
14. Suppliers to your industry; note movement and reasons.

Competitor data are the most difficult to obtain. In health care, regulations often require public notification of plans. This factor often makes competitive monitoring easy. Managers must recognize that whenever a competitor changes its strategy, it has the effect of changing your clinic's strategy.

The competitor has possibly restructured the basis for competition or the perception of the market. Too often health providers ignore competition, but no market plan should be developed without addressing the issues in this section.

■ The Internal Assessment

The fourth component of the internal/external assessment is the internal analysis. The object of this review is to obtain a general understanding of the workings of the organization from key participants. As a first step, each participant should independently evaluate the program or clinic with the form provided in Exhibit 5–6.

Completed forms should be compared for consistency among group members. Areas of low satisfaction or inconsistency should be explored. Recognized weak points may be obvious to competitors as the positions where they can establish dominance. It is important to recognize that this tool is an internal assessment and may not necessarily reflect accurately the opinions which outside physicians, consumers, and other important users might have regarding the organization.

In addition to this form, a comprehensive review should include examination of several other issues:

1. What has been the historical purpose of your clinic?
2. How has the hospital changed over the past decade?
3. When and how was it organized?
4. What has been the nature of its growth?
5. What is the basic policy of the organization? Is it "health care," or is it "profit"?

These questions require an examination of the original purpose of the organization. This investigation can lead to a reexamination of the appropriateness of the original mission, in light of the competitive factors addressed in an earlier phase of the internal/external analysis.

Any marketing actions contemplated by a clinic will be affected by finances. A review of this functional area is a necessity.

6. What has been the financial history of the organization?
7. How has it been capitalized?
8. Have there been any accounts receivable problems?
9. What is the inventory investment?
10. How successful has the organization been with the various services promoted?
11. Is the total volume (gross revenue, utilization) increasing or decreasing?
12. Have there been any fluctuations in revenue? If so, what were they due to?

EXHIBIT 5-6
Overall Internal Assessment

	Internal Assessment					
	(check one) Satisfaction Three Years Ago			(check one) Satisfaction in Current Year		
	High	Med	Low	High	Med	Low
Outpatient utilization						
Inpatient census						
Age of medical staff						
Medical staff relations						
Quality of service						
Relationships with key regulatory agencies, e.g., HSA, rate commission						
Cost containment/effectiveness efforts						
Community support ("This is my hospital or clinic.")						
Level of community awareness						
Responsiveness to unmet health care needs in the community						
Employee relations						
Employee recruiting						
Share of market served						
Breadth of product line						
Organization objectives						
Compensation structure for employees						
Financial position of organization						
Technological capability						
Efficiency of organization in service delivery						
Investment intensity						
Vertical integration						

Conclusion:

The following seven questions require an honest and challenging investigation of the organization's strengths and weaknesses. A reputation as a major teaching hospital with excellent research capacity may not be a strength in establishing a primary care clinic. High prices might cause consumers to perceive the teaching hospital as appropriate only for "serious" illnesses, and would not be a competitive advantage.

What are the organization's present strengths and weaknesses in:

13. Managment capabilities?
14. Medical staff?
15. Technical facilities?
16. Reputation?

17. Financial capabilities?
18. Image?
19. Medical facilities?

The final three questions pertain to the personnel envirnoment of the organization. What is the labor environment for:

20. Medical staff (nurses, physicians, etc.)?
21. Support personnel?
22. How are weaknesses being compensated for and strengths being used?

■ The Marketing Function and Programs

The final step in the analysis of internal capability pertains directly to the marketing activities of the clinic or hospital. Before considering the specific strategies of the organization, the structure of its marketing responsibilities must be assessed.

1. Does the organization have a high-level marketing officer to analyze, plan, and implement its marketing work?
2. Are the other persons directly involved in marketing activity able people? Is there a need for more training, incentives, supervision, or evaluation?
3. Are the marketing responsibilities optimally structured to serve the needs of different activities, products, markets, and territories?
4. Does the organization's personnel understand and practice the marketing concept?

These questions provide an understanding of whether or not the functional arrangement of the marketing activity is appropriate. Implementation of action strategies requires control by an individual with responsibility and authority.

As any manager familiar with marketing knows, service, price, promotion, and distribution decisions are the core aspects of the marketing mix. Although inspection of each mix element in isolation is a part of the internal/external analysis, the overall marketing program should be reviewed.

5. What is the organization's core strategy for achieving its objectives, and is it likely to succeed?
6. Is the organization allocating enough resources (or too many) to accomplish its marketing tasks?
7. Are the marketing resources allocated optimally to the various markets, territories, and products of the organization?
8. Are the marketing resources allocated optimally to the major elements of the marketing mix; i.e., product quality, personal contact, promotion, and distribution?

The preceding questions focus on the organization's strategy and the resource allocation necessary to accomplish this strategy. Related consideration must be given to the implementation of the marketing program.

9. Does the organization develop an annual marketing plan? Is the planning procedure effective?
10. Does the organization implement control procedures (monthly, quarterly, etc.) to insure that its annual plan objectives are being achieved?
11. Does the organization carry out periodic studies to determine the contribution and effectiveness of various marketing activities?
12. Does the organization have an adequate marketing information system to service the needs of managers in planning and controlling various markets?

The remaining areas of the marketing analysis pertain to specific mix elements. Much of the data needed to complete the remaining portions of this task will be contained in internal records of the group or in management judgments.

Products/services. As marketing actions are prepared for the future planning period, a reanalysis of existing service strategies is warranted.

1. Complete a list of your organization's products and services, both present and proposed.
2. What are the general outstanding characteristics of each product or service?
3. What superiority or distinctiveness of products or services do you have, as compared to competing organizations?
      What are the weaknesses?
      Should any product be phased out?
      Should any product be added?
4. What is the total cost per serivce (in use)? Is the service over or under utilized?
5. What services are most heavily used? Why?
      Are there distinct groups of users?
      What is the profile of patients/physicians who use the services?
6. What are your organization's policies regarding:
      Number and types of services to offer?
      Assessing needs for service addition/deletion?
7. History of major products and services:
      How many did the organization originally have?
      How many have been added or dropped?
      What important changes have taken place in services during the last 10 years?
      Has demand for the services increased or decreased?
      What are the most common complaints against the service?

What services could be added to your organization that would make it more attractive to patients, medical staff, nonmedical personnel?

What are the strongest points of your services to patients, medical staff, nonmedical personnel?

8. Have you any other features that individualize your service or give you an advantage over competitors?

It is important for members of the analysis team to maintain a market perspective as they proceed through the questions. That is, in considering the advantages of a program, it must be done from the buyer's view, not the internal clinic or hospital perspective.

Pricing strategy. The importance of price need not be reviewed. Yet changing reimbursement structures and competitive trends requires a close reexamination of historical pricing practices. Internally, the rationale for existing prices and the external price trends should be reviewed.

1. What is the pricing strategy of the organization?
    Cost-plus.
    Return on investment.
    Stabilization.
    Demand.
2. How are prices for services determined?
    How often are prices reviewed?
    What factors contribute to price increase or decrease?
3. What have been the price trends for the past five years?

In addition, the organization must take into account market perceptions of price, as well as price elasticity. Although the common view is that prices must be lowered, one group practice conducted a study on its market's price sensitivity. Data revealed that area consumers expected to pay a higher charge for an office visit than the group's present price level.

4. How are your pricing policies viewed by:
    Patients?
    Physicians?
    Third-party payers?
    Competitors?
    Regulators?
5. How are price promotions used?
6. What would be the impact of a higher or lower price on demand?

Promotional strategy. The promotional strategy of an organization consists of personal selling, advertising, and public relations. Salespeople often are used by multispecialty clinics to aid outreach efforts, or by hospitals for industrial health programs. Compensation, sales force size, and account allocation should be periodically examined.

1. Is the sales force large enough to accomplish the organization's objectives?
2. Is the sales force organized along the proper principles of specialization (territory, market, product)?
3. Does the sales force show high morale, ability, and effort? Is it sufficiently trained and motivated?
4. Are the procedures adequate for setting quotas and evaluating performance?

Recently the advertising component of promotion has received greater attention by health care organizations. Central to a review of advertising is campaign focus.

5. What is the purpose of the organization's present promotional activities (including advertising)?
    Protective
    Educational.
    Search out new markets.
    Develop all markets.
    Establish a new service.
6. Has this purpose undergone any change in recent years?
7. To whom has advertising been largely directed:
    Donors?
    Patients?
        Former.
        Current.
        Prospective.
    Physicians?
        On staff.
        Potential.

Media strategy should be evaluated periodically.

8. Is the cost per thousand still favorable?
9. Is it delivering the desired audience?
10. What media have been used?
11. Are the media still effective in reaching the intended audience?

The final concerns are those of copy strategy and periodic evaluation of advertising.

12. Are the objectives (reviewed in Question 5) being met?
13. What copy appeals have been notable in terms of response?
14. What methods have been used for measuring advertising effectiveness?

Public relations.   Public relations is a common promotional tool for health providers. Yet this function also requires a periodic analysis to retain its value.

1. What is the role of public relations?
    Is it a separate function/department?
    What is its scope of responsibilities?
2. Has the public relations effort led to regular coverage?
3. Are the public relations objectives integrated with the overall promotional plan?

This last question is of particular importance. Advertising and public relations are often the responsibilities of different people within a hospital. Therefore, a structure must be established to integrate the objectives of each activity. In this way the organization can benefit from the synergistic effect of integrated actions. A final question pertains to the assessment of effectiveness.

4. Are procedures established and used to measure the results from the public relations program?

Distribution strategies.   The final component of the marketing analysis pertains to distribution. How are services delivered or provided to the market?

1. What are the distribution trends in the industry?
    What services are being performed on an outpatient basis?
    What services are being performed on an at-home basis?
    Are satellite facilities being used?
2. What factors are considered in location decisions?
3. How important is distribution in establishing a competitive advantage for a particular service?
    Where does the hospital or clinic stand on this component?

■ Summary

The internal/external analysis is a comprehensive look at the external and internal factors which may affect marketing decisions. Not every question presented in the previous sections can or will be answered in the depth desired by all key management personnel. However, a major outcome of the process is to force introspection regarding management's views and the organization's position. Large and small organizations should attempt some level of environmental analysis. Recognizing that the small group practice could not implement the detailed analysis reviewed here, Exhibit 5–7 presents a brief overview analysis as a complement.

In completing this abbreviated form, the questions posed in the more detailed analysis can be used as guidelines. Appendix A contains a complete

EXHIBIT 5–7
Brief Overview Analysis

I. Market Environment Review
  A. Markets
    1. Who are your major markets and publics (i.e., who are you serving now)? List in order of importance and indicate the percentage of your total business that each market represents. How will this look five years from now?
  B. Customer Satisfaction and Needs
    1. What is your position in these markets (i.e., MDs, patients)? List positives and negatives in short phrases.
  C. Competition
    1. Who is your major competitor? If more than one, list in order of significance to you. What advantages do they have?
  D. External Environment
    1. What trends or developments are currently taking place that will affect (positively and negatively) your ability to market your products?

II. Market System Review
  A. Program Objectives
    1. State your program objectives. List with expected outcomes and methods of measurement.
    2. If you were required to reduce your financial resources by 30 percent, how would you allocate your resources?
  B. Marketing Mix
    1. What is the basic strategy for achieving the program's current objective (e.g., diversify, specialize, increase medical staff, encourage more physician participation, attract different kinds of employees, etc.)?
    2. How would you be affected by changes in the following?
      a. Pricing
      b. Promotion
      c. Distribution
      d. Products

III. Detailed Marketing Activity Review
  A. Products: What needs do they meet? What is your competitive advantage?
  B. Price:
    1. How are prices set? Describe current pricing policy. Please comment on the following factors:
      a. Relationship to cost
      b. Impact of competition
      c. Reimbursement implications
      d. Physician relationships
      e. Other
  C. Distribution: What alternatives exist?
  D. Promotion: What is your competitive strategy?
  E. Detail your volume and profitability over the last five years.

list of the questions posed within this chapter for a complete internal/external analysis.

At several points in this analysis, information gaps become apparent. For example, the hospital may not have real measures of the organization's image in various markets. Marketing research may be required to obtain the needed data. Specific marketing research methodologies are beyond the scope of this book. However, Appendix B contains a review of the more common data collection methodologies. After completing the internal/external analysis, recognition of the organization's existing market position and how it was achieved should be realized. Moving to strategy formulation is then possible.

References

Berkowitz, Eric N., and William A. Flexner. "The Marketing Audit: A Tool for Health Service Organizations." *Health Care Management Review,* Fall 1978, pp. 51–57.

Cannon, J. Thomas. "Auditing the Competitive Environment." In *Concepts of Corporate Strategy,* ed. John W. Bonge and Bruce P. Coleman. New York: Macmillan, 1972.

King, William R., and David L. Cleland. "Environment Information Systems for Strategic Marketing Planning." *Journal of Marketing,* October 1974.

Oxenfeldt, A. R., "The Marketing Audit as a Total Evaluation Program." In *Analyzing and Improving Marketing Performance, Report No. 32.* New York: American Management Association, 1959, p. 26.

Shuchman, A., "The Marketing Audit: Its Nature, Purposes, and Problems." In *Analyzing and Improving Marketing Performance, Report No. 32.* New York: American Management Association, 1959, p. 13.

CHAPTER 6

THE STRATEGY ACTION MATCH —STEP 3

Step 3: Strategy Action Match and Setting Marketing Objectives

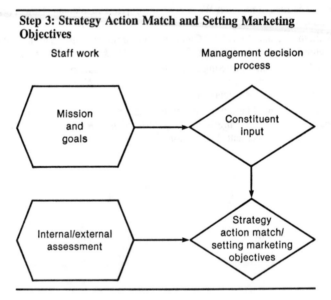

Several alternative models have been advanced by management experts to help businesses conceptualize problems related to mission, growth, and competition. One widely cited model was developed by the Boston Consulting Group (BCG). The BCG matrix was designed to look at a portfolio or group of products in a company. The areas in which the portfolio is evaluated are a product's market share and growth in the overall market. Exhibit 6–1 shows the BCG matrix and the alternatives within which to plot products or services.

EXHIBIT 6–1
The BCG Matrix

The matrix
Market share

	High	Low
High	★ Star	? Problem child
Low	$ Cash cow	— Dog

(Growth: High / Low on vertical axis)

Source: Reprinted from Bruce Henderson, *Henderson on Corporate Strategy* (Cambridge, Mass.: Abt Books, 1979). By permission of the publisher, © 1979.

The objective in using this matrix is to identify and eliminate poor performance areas (dogs), and to generate business opportunities which have high growth in growing markets (stars). The model depends heavily on the notions of relative market share and growth. These concepts, although directly relevant in manufacturing firms, are often less pertinent in service businesses. Growth in market share in manufacturing often means greater efficiency, lower unit cost, and greater profit. In service businesses, with personnel directly involved in each sale (or interaction), efficiency with growth may or may not occur.

An alternative matrix is the General Electric model, which evaluates *industry attractiveness* and *business strengths*. In this method, as illustrated in Exhibit 6–2, factors relating to industry attractiveness include: industry growth, vulnerability to new competitors, profitability, and competitive intensity. Business strengths relate to factors such as: Do we have capability and experience in this business? Does it allow for integration within the company? Does it make us more productive? Is it of value to the firm? The goal of this method is to find those businesses and services which show the greatest promise for the organization. Both models are useful in making decisions about new business and investment opportunities, but what about hospitals and other health care services that are already in business? What about health care organizations which are committed by mission to a service or location, regardless of what BCG or the G.E. model might indicate?

One model which helps a business identify strategy *within the current business* was developed by the Management Analysis Center (MAC) Inc. and is called the *Retail Positioning Map*. This model concentrates less on what is the best, new business, and more on what to do with the existing business. Exhibit 6–3 provides the matrix model used by MAC. It involves two dimensions—a value-added dimension and a breadth-of-product-line dimension.

The term, *value-added*, refers to items such as hours of service, loca-

70

EXHIBIT 6–2
G.E. Stoplight Model

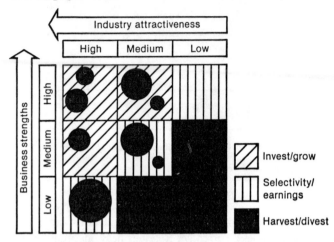

Source: Reprinted from *Maintaining Strategies for the Future Through Current Crises* (Fairfield, Conn.: General Electric Co., 1975), with permission of the publisher, © 1975.

EXHIBIT 6–3
Retail Positioning Map: Four Star Matrix

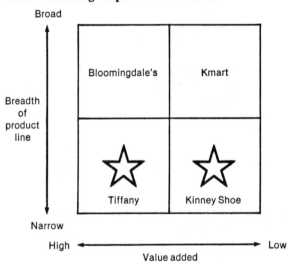

Source: Reprinted from William T. Gregor and Eileen M. Friars, *"Money Merchandising,"* a report prepared by the Management Analysis Center (MAC) Inc., 1983, with permission of the publisher, © 1983.

tion, credit policy, prestige, schedule system, phone call follow-up performance, and other factors that tend to differentiate one service from another.
Breadth of product lines describes the number of services available, such as
a large, multispecialty group as opposed to a five-person, single specialty/
internal medicine clinic.

Bloomingdale's, for example, has a wide product line with an extensive value-added dimension in the areas of credit options, store locations,
credit policy, prestige, and personal service. Kmart also has a broad product
line but few "extras." Tiffany, on the other hand, is narrow in product line
but specializes in several value-added features. Kinney Shoes is narrow both
in product line and value-added features.

Whereas each organization tries to build a loyal base of customers,
they do so in different ways, including large operations versus small, and
specialty operations versus nonspecialty. Each method creates a differential
advantage between competitors for a specific customer group. This strategy
also suggests that success may lie in not being like everyone else. Instead of
having a routine hospital emergency room, it may be possible to develop a
different, value-added service in order to be set apart from the competition.
Sony, for example, decided to compete in a new radio market so it created
the Walkman radio. Savin wanted to compete in a different copier market so
it went to the inexpensive market using a dealer network. Health care organizations can also compete differently, often by changing the game rules and
creating new ideas to meet market demand. For example, a physician
housecall service may allow for competition on an access dimension. (That
is, by being more available to the patient.)

The MAC model suggests that an organization may, by mission,
choose to be in the hospital business, but within that business a hospital can
select how and within which areas to compete. For example, most hospitals
in a community may rush to be a Bloomingdale's of health care, offering
much value-added service in all specialties. However, with the competition
rushing to this strategy, several alternative and profitable options could be
available Exhibit 6–4 shows examples of alternatives to the Bloomingdale's
(Mayo) strategy: a narrow breadth of product line and a high value-added
dimension such as Boston Children's Hospital, or low value-added and narrow product line such as an internal medicine practice, or a low value-added
and broad product line such as a low-cost hospital. A hospital or clinic has an
opportunity to select market segments that it would like to attract, and therefore, it designs a package of value-added services and a range of products to
appeal to targeted markets. This is often called *field positioning*.

Field positioning describes the basis on which a service competes. The
elements include selecting target market segments and services to be included in the value-added package. Field positioning involves a variety of
strategic decisions. These decisions include: how broad or narrow the service
line should be, in which segment or segments to compete, which services to

EXHIBIT 6–4
Positioning Map: Four-Star Matrix

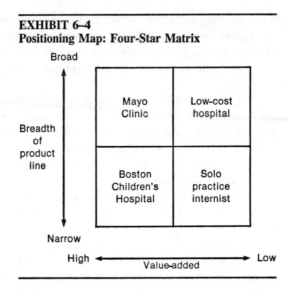

add to the package to make it attractive to a segment, and where to act against the competition. For example, a narrow focus in a specific market segment with a specific specialty would be geriatrics. This is a service offered to a single target. A broad focus would be a medical group organized to make house calls. In this case, the group would cater to old and middle-aged, homebound people. The services would also include a broad package of medical care support with value-added services including convenience—the actual house call. The idea is not to try to play the field, but to be able to select which markets to capture, and where and how to compete by selecting a value-added package and product line.

All of the alternative models described aid in developing strategic thinking. They help to develop ideas regarding opportunities and problems. One of the difficulties with the models, however, is that they talk either about what business to be in or not to be in, or what to do within a given business, but not both. The connection between choosing the right business area and what to do within that area is an important match. Yet it is a match which, until now, has not often been adequately developed by hospital or clinic leadership. This chapter will provide a useful model that helps determine what business to be in *and* what to do in each business. This process is called the *strategy action match*.

The focus of this match is on the concept of a product life cycle for services. Few concepts in marketing have received such attention. Several attempts at modeling the curve have been made for consumer durables,[1]

---

[1]Frank Bass, "A New Product Growth Model for Consumer Durables," *Management Science* 15 (January 1969), pp. 215–27; Stephen G. Harrell and Elmer D. Taylor, "Modeling the Product Life Cycle for Consumer Durables," *Journal of Marketing* 45 (Fall 1981), pp. 65–75.

technological innovations[2] and new product formulations.[3] Although admonitions have existed to forget this concept,[4] recent writers have observed that research on life cycles in the marketing literature do not support this conclusion.[5] One author has suggested that "the most fundamental variable in determining an appropriate strategy is the stage of the product life cycle."[6] A comprehensive list of suggested additional references on the life cycle concept is presented at the end of this chapter. One author has summarized the life cycle concept as a versatile framework for appropriate strategy alternatives and an aid to directing management attention toward the underlying dynamics of a competitive market.[7] In this book, the life cycle concept serves as the normative model by which health care managers focus on their internal strategies relative to the external competitive market.

The strategy action match is based on a careful analysis of both marketplace conditions and the position of a specific service within that marketplace, using the data obtained in Chapter 5. The theory of the product life cycle is useful in conducting this analysis.

Life cycle analysis is based on the notion that products, services, and even entire markets all have a life cycle. Exhibit 6–5 shows the typical life cycle curve with its four stages of activity. The horizontal line represents time. Time could be a matter of months or many years. The vertical line represents growth over time, from one year to the next or one month to the next. Growth might be in terms of sales, revenue, or patient days. Within this chart, four life cycle stages are plotted.

Introduction. This is when a new product or service is first brought to market. Sales and revenue are slow. By and large, the market is unaware of the product offering. For example, the first urgent care service opens in the community. The curve slowly rises as more people become aware of the facility and how it can be used.

Growth. Demand begins to grow and the size of the total market expands. Often, a competitor enters the market, and people become more aware of the urgent care facilities. Both competitors promote their services, and there is a synergistic effect on the market.

---

[2]Frank Bass, "The Relationship Between Diffusion Rates, Experience Curves, and Demand Elasticities for Consumer Durable Technological Innovations," *Journal of Business* 53 (1980), pp. 551–67; Douglas Tigert and Behrooz Farivar, "The Bass New Product Growth Model: A Sensitivity Anaysis For a High Technology Product," *Journal of Marketing* 45 (Fall 1981), pp. 81–90.

[3]Harrell and Taylor, "Modeling the Product Life Cycle."

[4]N. Dhalla and S. Yuspeh, "Forget the Product Life Cycle," *Harvard Business Review* 54 (January–February 1976), pp. 102–12.

[5]Hans B. Thorelli and Stephen G. Burnett, "The Nature of Product Life Cycles for Industrial Goods Businesses," *Journal of Marketing* 45 (Fall 1981), pp. 97–108.

[6]C. W. Hofer, "Toward a Contingency Theory of Business Strategy," *Academy of Management Journal* 18 (Decmber 1975), p. 798.

[7]George Day, "The Product Life Cycle; Analysis and Application Issues," *Journal of Marketing* 45 (Fall 1981), pp. 60–67.

EXHIBIT 6–5
The Product Life Cycle

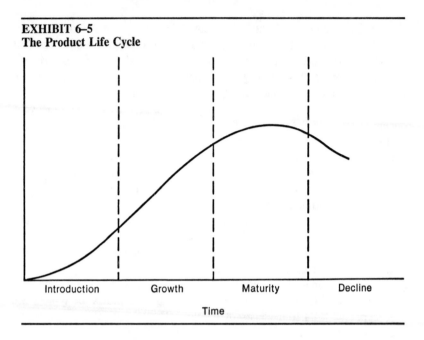

Maturity. Demand levels off. A slight increase occurs as the last potential buyers in the market finally utilize the urgent care facility, and loyal buyers continue to return at their average utilization level. Maturity can occur for several reasons, however, other than saturation. Because of demographics, for example, pediatrics is in the mature stage as the population ages.

Decline. The service begins to lose appeal, and sales drift downward. Most likely some new health care alternative has started.

It is important to recognize that some products, such as Pet Rocks or first-generation CT scanners, go through the life cycle quickly. Others go through at a much slower rate such as railroads, tuberculosis hospitals, polio treatment, and some respiratory therapy treatments. Still others seem to run through the life cycle only to recover again, as did Arm & Hammer baking soda. This is done through the application of new uses, which point out opportunities to use the product for brushing teeth, as a refrigerator freshener, or as a carpet deodorizer. A similar example is mental health, which has matured on an inpatient basis, while a new growth life cycle is occurring with outpatient mental health programs.

Life cycle is a very useful concept. It helps managers anticipate what is likely to happen in the future, including information about when competitors may enter the arena. Insights regarding the occurrence of pricing changes are also provided. In addition, life cycle analysis underscores the fact that new products and services are constantly being developed, causing other products and services to decline over time. (See Exhibit 6–6.)

This concept is useful for specific products and services and for entire

EXHIBIT 6–6
Impact of New Services

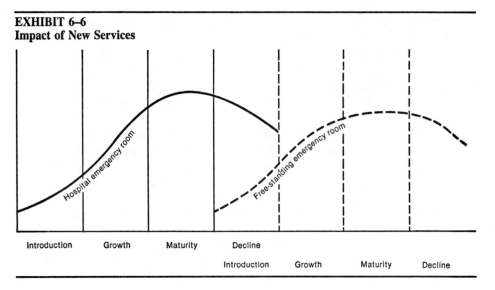

Introduction	Growth	Maturity	Decline			
			Introduction	Growth	Maturity	Decline

product categories. For example, the entire tuberculosis hospital industry went through the life cycle. In many large cities, the entire hospital industry of the community may be in the maturing phase as ambulatory care, urgent care, PPOs, HMOs, and private review establish new life cycles at the introductory stage. Listed below are the four stages of the *marketplace* life cycle. This refers to the monitoring of the service within the market area, as opposed to the life cycle of the organization's which was discussed previously.

Introduction. This is the stage at which the service offering is first introduced into the market area.

Growth. The appearance of a competitor, as well as a rapid increase in the rate of patient volume, signals the second stage. Providers also begin to allocate more resources to this service.

Maturity. For most services, review begins to level off at some point in time. This result typically signals the onset of the maturity phase. Often at this point, some providers of the service will begin to drop the offering.

Decline. An ongoing decrease in revenue signals the onset of the fourth stage. Externally, competitors may have left the market as new services, or technological advances, replace the function of the existing service.

In many cases, it is difficult for a specific product or service to perform much differently from the entire market in which it is competing. For example, on the average, all domestic car manufacturers tend either to do well or perform badly as a group. Real estate companies are up or down as a group. Hospital use is often up or down as an industry. Medical supply sales are up or down as a group. Within these general ups and downs, some specific companies will do better than others, or at least not suffer the sales variations as much as their competitors do.

Assume five clinics exist in a given suburb and that they offer the same type of service to the community. Also assume that business is down an average of 10 percent in all five clinics. Unless a new service is developed or new market segment found, it is unreasonable to expect one clinic to outperform another.

When looking at the marketplace life cycle, it is important to compare a service to that of new competitors. The urgent care market is different (with a different life cycle) from the family practice life cycle. The PPO life cycle may be different from the HMO life cycle. Within each of these broad categories, it is likely that each service will have its own life cycle, as indicated by Exhibit 6–7. Studies have shown several variations to the product life cycle.[8]

In examining the life cycle charts of Exhibit 6–7, a noticeable difference can be observed in the introduction stage of the life cycle. For the urgent care concept, the introduction stage is relatively short. A health care organization entering this market must prepare for the entry of new competitors within a short time. A key goal may be to have as many sites as possible to block new competitors. This life cycle for urgent care, however, is very different from the PPO marketplace curve. In this scenario, an extended introduction stage is predicted. The health care organization entering this market must recognize the need for extended promotion. A longer than average time may be needed to educate the buyer regarding the benefits of this alternative program. Each service has an alternative shape to its life cycle curve. While no exact method exists for forecasting these shapes, managers must be sensitive to the possibility of a variation to the curve used in this chapter.

■ Organization versus Marketplace Life Cycle

The *strategy action match* is designed to: (1) match an organization's service's life cycle with the market place life cycle, and (2) determine what marketing planning strategies would be appropriate based on this match. In order to do the strategy action match, it is necessary to look at two life cycles: first, the specific service life cycle and second, the marketplace life cycle. The strategy matrix is essentially an overlapping of the organization life cycle (OLC) and market life cycle (MLC). Too often, managers view their own service's life in isolation, without considering the marketplace's life cycle. For example, a hospital introduced a pediatric service 10 years ago, and over the past 7 years has realized a small but increasing rate of growth. Often, these facts would lead to an increase in resources to the

---

[8]D. R. Rink and J. E. Swan, "Product Life Cycle Research: A Literature Review," *Journal of Business Research* 7 (September 1979), pp. 219–42.

EXHIBIT 6–7
Possible Alternative Life Cycles

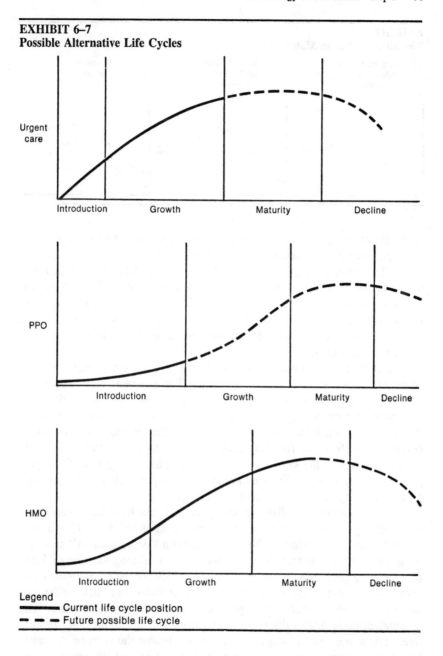

Legend
━━━━ Current life cycle position
━ ━ ━ Future possible life cycle

pediatric service. However, examination of the MLC in relation to the OLC leads to a different strategy guideline. During the past two years, two hospitals in the same metropolitan area dropped their pediatric service. The demographic profile of the community shows a rapidly aging population. The alternative suggestion, considering both factors, suggests that the organiza-

EXHIBIT 6–8
The Strategy Action Match Logic

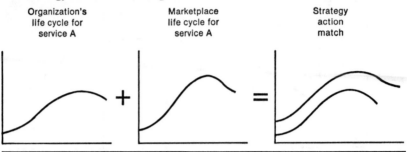

Organization's life cycle for service A	Marketplace life cycle for service A	Strategy action match

tion harvest this service and explore new opportunities. Exhibit 6–8 shows the logic used in the strategy action match.

The organization's service is plotted on its life cycle curve (OLC), and the marketplace is plotted on an industrywide curve (MLC). When looked at in combination, a strategic match is made. From this match is is possible to begin to make strategy and action decisions. Several combinations between the two curves can develop. Each combination results in different strategy and action decisions.

Exhibit 6–9 is an example of comparing the OLC for a specific service to the MLC for service at one point in time. The manager determines where the service (or program) is on the organization life cycle and the marketplace life cycle. For example, the Hunter Clinic has introduced a walk-in mammography screening program. The clinic is in the introduction stage of its organization life cycle for this service. Two competing facilities in town have been offering the same service for six months. Acceptance of this program is rapidly growing. From a market life cycle perspective, the mammography screening service is in the growth stage.

It is important to realize that an organization can be in a different phase of the life cycle than the market. An examination of Exhibit 6–10, on page 80, indicates that the Hunter Clinic must select a "differentiation" strategy. As a later entry to the market, the Hunter clinic's offering must be different than existing programs or the marketplace will view their program as just another alternative. Little incentive will exist for buyers to switch, or for new buyers to see the Hunter clinic's program as a more valuable offering. The remainder of this chapter discusses this strategy, along with the other alternatives. The major requirement in successfully selecting the appropriate strategies is the determination of the organization and market life cycle stages. Data generated through the internal and external assessments in Chapter 5 is essential for this process.

The strategy action matrix is presented in Exhibit 6–10. Its usefulness is determined by a manager's recognition of the organization's position on its OLC and the market's position on the MLC.

EXHIBIT 6–9
The Hunter Clinic Organizational Life Cycle for Mammography

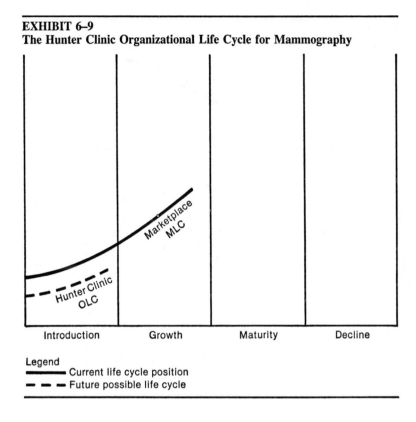

Introduction   Growth   Maturity   Decline

Legend
━━━━━ Current life cycle position
━ ━ ━ Future possible life cycle

Plotting the OLC and MLC will result in the formation of the strategy alternatives. The alternatives presented in this matrix are not all-inclusive, yet they provide directions for strategy formulation. The situation analysis should aid the manager in positioning the service offering on the matrix.

Each strategy guide is discussed in greater detail in the following section.

■ Strategy Options

"Go for It" Strategy

This strategy option occurs when a service is at the stage of new introduction, and the overall market demand is just beginning. This is a period characterized by few (or no) competitors. And two rather dramatic options—boom or bust—exist. It is possible that the market may never fully develop beyond this stage. Or the market may become strong, in which case a new service may be able to perform in a dramatic fashion.

If an organization is in a life cycle match position which indicates a

EXHIBIT 6–10
Strategy Action Match Matrix

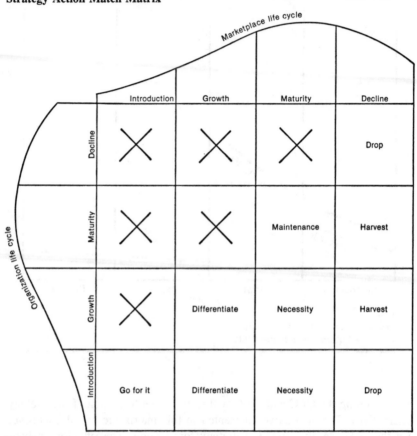

Legend
x = Position can not occur

"go for it" strategy, the key is to obtain strong marketplace recognition. In health care settings, because this recognition often relates to quality, it is necessary to maintain tight quality control at the "go for it" stage.

Each element of the marketing mix is used to maintain a competitive position at the "go for it" stage.

1. *The Product/Service.* For this element, the goal is to:
   a. Obtain service leadership by being one of the earliest organizations (if not the first) to introduce the service.
   b. Limit your service or product variations and reserve the introduction of options for a later time. Limiting the variations of your product offering is also a useful technique for four reasons.

EXHIBIT 6–11
"Go for It" Strategy

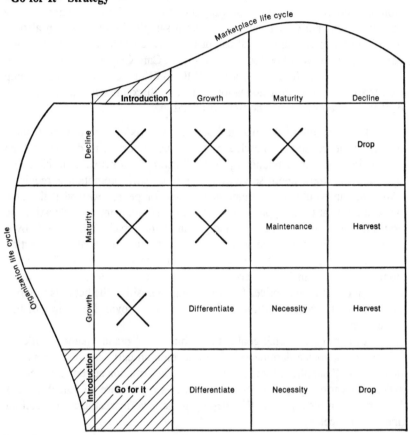

Legend
x = Position can not occur

It allows you to concentrate your resources on one option and develop a consistent quality service. Recall in Chapter 5 (Exhibit 5–6), an internal assessment regarding the organization's quality was completed. A critical review of these results is important before entering the "go-for it" stage.

It allows you to obtain recognition in the marketplace for a specific service.

It allows you to have new ideas or service modification for the time when you need to be more competitive.

It keeps your ideas confidential until it is necessary to introduce them for competitive advantage.

c. Carefully control quality.

2. *Price.* At the "go for it" position, a high-price strategy is often used because of a lack of competition and the need to recover the high front-end costs of setting up the program. Since a high-price strategy may inhibit customer use, it is suggested that a sample discount system also be used in order to encourage trial use or to increase consumer product knowledge. Examples would be for the new Urgent Care Center to give free blood pressure checks at the clinic, for the HMO to offer free preschool screening exams, or for the Health Education Center to discount seminars by 10 percent if two people from a household attend.

3. *Promotion.* When a new service is introduced in a market, there is often little consumer knowledge. It is thus important to develop a high advertising and public relations profile. Since the marketplace in this situation does not know about services of this type, such promotion is required. (An example would be free emergency kits for people who visit the new walk-in clinic at the shopping mall.) Promotional goals include educating the consumer about product benefits and gaining widespread marketplace knowledge of the existence of the service. In the long run, the goal is to position products and services that provide unique benefits to customers. These positioning benefits can include convenience, speed of service, better technology, or more attractive price. It is important to position the benefits in terms of the market's needs. Exhibit 5–2 of Chapter 5 provided a review of this dimension.

A major promotional goal is to establish the "brand" name in order to achieve marketplace dominance and to develop an early competitive advantage as "the" supplier of this service. Public information advertising, feature articles in various publications, and TV news reports are all valuable ways for services in the "go for it" category to achieve marketplace recognition and dominance.

4. *Distribution.* Strategies of distribution relate to the alternative ways of providing the service to customers. At this stage, however, very tight control should be placed on distribution. The most accepted model is to limit the use of any distribution system to those over which you have total control. In this way, quality and performance problems can be completely worked out, and the product will be provided as intended. If a complex distribution network, such as franchises or outreach clinics, is developed too early (before product problems and systems have been worked out), it becomes difficult to manage. Once all "systems" are smooth, "go for it." Then move as quickly as possible to establish a distribution system that provides the greatest possible market penetration.

The Differentiation Strategy

This strategy occurs at two points of the strategy action match—the intro-growth and the growth-growth stages. In both situations, the major need of the organization is for differentiation from its competitors, and an organiza-

EXHIBIT 6–12
Differentiation Strategy—Scenario 1

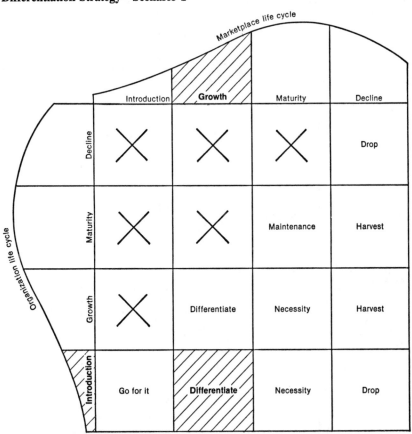

Legend
x = Position can not occur

tion's concern is to establish a differential competitive advantage. In considering a basis for differentiation, Exhibits 5–4 and 5–5 of Chapter 5 are valuable. These analyses require a consideration of competitors' strengths and weaknesses. Also, a major focus of these audits is to determine the basis for competition. Differentiation may be developed around the competitive profile. Before discussing the range of strategy options, consider two scenarios for each condition.

Scenario 1: Organization-intro/marketplace-growth. In this scenario, your service is being introduced, although offerings of a similar nature already exist in the marketplace. In Dallas, for example, one clinic has opened an Urgi-Center as a low-cost alternative to the hospital emergency room, and an extended-hours source of care after normal physicians' office hours.

EXHIBIT 6–13
Differentiation Strategy—Scenario 2

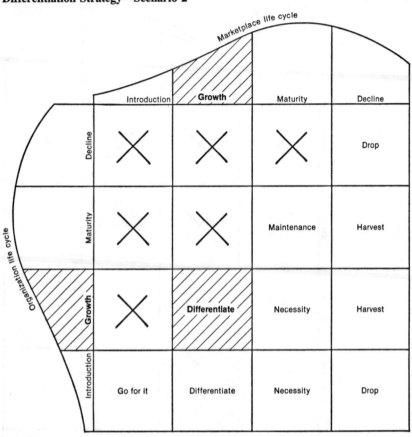

Legend
x = Position can not occur

This facility has been open for one year. Your group is now about to open a similar clinic. The market has been growing, but your group is just entering. What strategies should be implemented?

Scenario 2: Organization-growth/marketplace-growth. In this condition, you were one of the first hospitals to introduce a sports medicine program. Soon after your service introduction, two other hospitals entered the market with similar services. People in the community are now aware of such services, and demand is growing for you and your competitors. What is your next move?

Differentiation. In either scenario, the differentiation strategy is important. All elements of the marketing mix should be directed to the differentiation of your organization from its competitors. Consider the variations:

1. *Product.* In the differentiation strategy, consider creating a more segmented service offering. That is, the sports medicine program can be segmented by age of the potential user. Develop a program for teens and preteens. Establish links with park sports leagues, high school coaches, or parents. Creating a version for a specific age group will provide a more dominant image within each segment and allow for differentiation from competitors' general programs. These segments should be selected as a function of their size, needs, and the organization's ability to meet those needs. In Chapter 5, assessment was required in Exhibits 5–1 and 5–2, on the size and segment need issues. Exhibit 5–3 of Chapter 5 considers the internal ability of the professional staff to respond to those segment demands.

2. *Pricing.* Price can be viewed as a very successful differentiating tactic. Matched with program (i.e., product) variations, the organization can create different versions of the same clinical service. For example, create a sports medicine package. Fees for medical service can include rehabilitation at a number of community health clubs. Or in obstetrics, whereas natural birthing programs are the norm, offer package pricing for prenatal to postnatal checkups. Price variations can be made to broaden the appeal of the service offering beyond the original market in which competition is presently occurring.

3. *Promotion.* The promotion element plays an important role in aiding differentiation. In the "go for it" stage, advertising is needed to create awareness. In the differentiation stage, *ad copy must shift from awareness to trial of your service.* The need, in this phase, is to create preference among buyers. This strategy must be coordinated with changes in the other elements of the mix. That is, now is the time to focus on *longer hours, lower prices, more specialized services, and a more comprehensive program.*

Promotional programs, such as giving away free emergency kits (used in the "go for it" stage), assume less importance in this scenario. While promotion is important in other strategy action positions, at the organizational growth/market growth match, awareness of the offering already exists. The need is to encourage the market to use your service rather than a competitor's offering. This must be done by concentrating on the advantages of the service, rather than by informing buyers that the service exists.

The sales force role often becomes more important at this stage. The key goal for your sales staff is to lockup the channels of distribution. If a company is going to go with just one alcohol/chemical dependency program, the contract must be signed with your group. Likewise, a sales effort may be needed in any situation in which the buyer has more than one offering from which to choose.

4. *Distribution.* This element of the marketing mix is the most common way for health care services to achieve differentiation. In order to distinguish your service offering from that of competitors, consideration should be given to:

Hours/days of availability.

Number of site locations.

Accessibility/convenience.

Manner in which service is distributed.

For many organizations, the approach to differentiation is to provide more intensive distribution (i.e., multiple site locations and longer hours). A scenario regarding Urgi-Centers was presented earlier in the discussion of the organization-intro/market-growth match. The best form of differentiation here might be a number of Urgi-Center sites, with one brand name, throughout the Dallas area.

Necessity Strategy

This type of strategy occurs when the market is mature. An organization may just have introduced this service or be in the growth stage. This strategy is carried out in the belief that this service is needed to effectively compete, even when it is known that the service may not gain a large share of the existing market. The only limitation to capturing this share is the prior existence of competitors.

Consider this common scenario:

In Engertown, several clinics have offered family practitioners for primary care needs. The Maxwell Clinic has offered specialty care services for 20 years. Five years ago, the physicians at the Maxwell Clinic finally decided to enter the primary care end of medicine to ensure a referral base. Three family practitioners were brought into the group. Although the Maxwell Clinic was a late entry into this service in Engertown, a community with a stable population, the demand for family practitioners within the clinic is still growing.

Although it is recognized that achievement in this scenario will be difficult, possible gains can be realized. One approach is to position this late entry against the leading competitor. The need is to differentiate. An alternative option is to select a market segment that may have special needs and develop the service to meet those needs. This will help to develop reputation, cost control, and recognized community capability.

Each element of the marketing mix is important for a successful necessity strategy.

1. *Product.* Because the organization is entering the market late with its own offering, the expectations of the service already exist in the market. Any *necessity* service offering must be at least equal to those of relevant competitors. A potential for profit can result if the late-entry service is more closely tailored to a specific market segment. For example, in one community the physicians in gynecology have had established practices. A new OB/GYN service is opened. It has a supervised child care area staffed by college students majoring in child development. Because of this service, a

EXHIBIT 6–14
Necessity Strategy

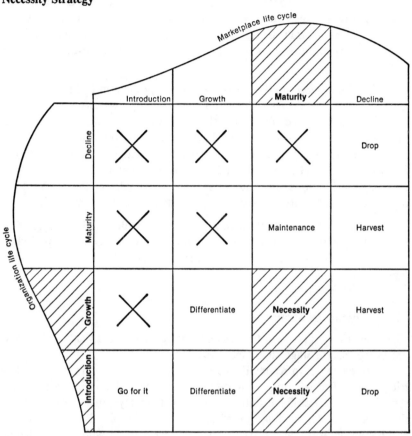

Legend
x = Position can not occur

woman can bring her child with her to the doctor, and while she has her exam, the child has supervised play activities. This late entry to the single-parent, female household market might be a desirable feature to shift share from existing providers.

2. *Price.* To a great extent, price is not a variable which the organization has in its control under a necessity strategy. Usually the buyers have expectations or knowledge of existing price options because the existing competitive entries have established the viable price ranges.

The Howard Hospital has decided it must offer health education courses. In the community, there are two ranges of prices for weight control programs. Some groups offer a high-price option with medical, psychological, and nutrition staff interaction. On the other end are very low-cost lecture programs. Since Howard Hospital is a late entry in this market, it decides to offer a middle-price program. The marketplace is mature and thus aware of the alternatives. This late offering will probably be viewed as an "expensive" low-end program or a "cheap" premium program. In the necessity stage, the organization must recognize the existing price structure for the service.

3. *Promotion.* In the necessity strategy promotion is difficult. Often the program is introduced at this late stage to keep physicians at the hospital or patients at the clinic. Promotion should be on a mass basis to inform the market that there is no need to look elsewhere. (You, too, offer the service.)

If, in the necessity stage, the organization decides to focus on a market segment, a personal sales effort may be more important. A key goal is to encourage switching to the late entry. A personal sales contact may be required to encourage trial by explaining the unique service benefits.

4. *Distribution.* Distribution plays a small role in this strategy. The need is to match the competition. If the market segment can be appealed to for a distribution requirement, then this is the focus of a competitive advantage.

The Maintenance Strategy

This scenario occurs when the organization life cycle and market life cycle are in the mature stage simultaneously.

For example, in Knoxville there are six hospitals which provide pediatric service. The last hospital to add such a service did so in 1968. While there have been occasional shifts of relative patient days, most hospitals view this area as stable, heading toward decline. Your hospital has maintained a steady census in pediatrics. The question is what to do with this service in the next five-year planning period.

The maintenance strategy suggests just that—keep what you've got. Occasionally organizations attempt to gain share or revenue in this stage. Yet the incremental cost of each patient day may not equal the marginal revenue. It is probably not cost-efficient to go to the expense of encouraging physicians to shift patients to you in order to get the additional patient days in the mature stage. In following the maintenance strategy, the assumption is that the level of maturity is satisfactory. (If not, move to "Drop Strategy" discussion.)

1. *Product.* In the maintenance strategy, the product must be reexamined in order for the organization to stay alive. Often the leader in a mature business notices a loss of business. Competitors have begun to attract smaller market niches which once represented your target market. A reexamination of the service is necessary to explore opportunities to gain back prior users or to reposition your service against that of competitors.

EXHIBIT 6–15
Maintenance Strategy

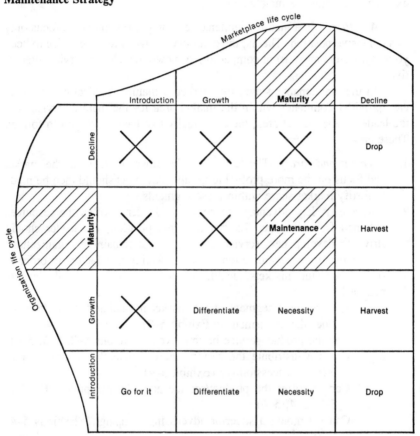

Legend
x = This position can not occur

2. *Promotion.* A key element of the maintenance strategy is promotion. The goal is to keep the users you presently have. Ongoing efforts to insure that patients return to your clinic and that physicians use your pediatric service are the goals. Post-use follow-up, through letters, phone calls, or sales force contact, is necessary to monitor the continuing satisfaction of your clientele. Newsletters, tie-in educational seminars, etc., also become important in keeping the loyalty base of your existing users.

3. *Distribution.* Distribution strategy is continued at its present level. Clinic hours or locations are changed only by necessity, that is, if a competitor offers night hours, a similar approach might have to be borrowed.

Because there are no new buyers entering the market in the mature stage, existing users must be maintained.

4. *Price*. In a mature maintenance strategy, pricing is the focus only as a defensive position. That is, the common change is to lower price to keep your loyal users away from competitors or newly developed service alternatives.

In the maintenance stage, the market is mature. Typically one health care provider dominates within the market area for the mature service. For the leader in the market area, there are really two basic strategies to follow. These are:

1. *Segment and fortify*. The leader has the power to segment the market and focus on the more profitable groups. Attempts should then be made to fortify market share within these segments.
2. *Innovate*. A key advantage to being the leader is often the resources obtained from revenue. To maintain this position, the leader should strive to develop new service offerings. The remaining organizations must return to a reexamination of the marketing mix factors in order to survive in mature markets. Health care providers who are not the leaders must ask:

   Is there some segment of the market not being served? (Reconsider the assessment in Exhibit 5–2)

   Can the product/service be improved? (Exhibits 5–2, 5–3, 5–6)

   Can we distribute the service more efficiently or significantly increase accessibility? (Exhibit 5–4)

   Can we offer the product/service at a cheaper price? (Exhibits 5–3, 5–4, 5–6)

   Can we mount a superior advertising campaign? (Exhibits 5–4, 5–5)

This stage requires action. Increased sales and market share can only come from a competitor. A fight for share or a search for new alternatives become the only courses for growth.

Harvest Strategy

One of the most difficult decisions a health care manager faces is having to harvest (phase out) a service which no longer produces enough value to the organization. While it is possible that political and public relations pressure may cause an organization to avoid the harvest strategy, it is still an important option to consider in two cases: Organization-Growth/Market-Decline and Organization-Maturity/Market-Decline. In either case, the same strategy applies. If managed properly, the harvest strategy can be employed to maximize organizational effectiveness.

Organization-Growth/Market-Decline. In this scenario, your product is growing in a market which is declining. In other words, at the moment, you

EXHIBIT 6–16
Harvest Strategy

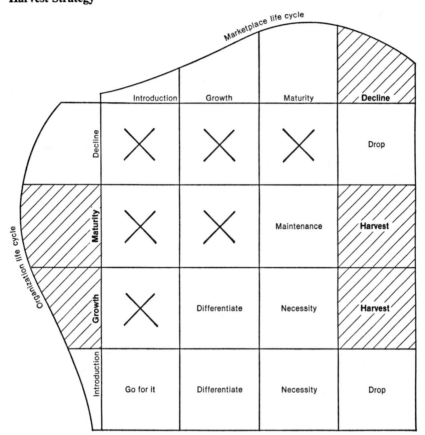

Legend
x = Position can not occur

are moving forward, and against the grain of the market. It is likely that your ability to maintain this pattern in the long run is remote, as the primary demand for the service is diminishing. As a result, the harvest strategy applies.

Organization-Maturity/Market-Decline. In this scenario, the logic of the harvest strategy is more obvious. Not only is your service not growing, but the entire market is in a stage of decline. By this point, the organization should be limiting its resources in this service or product line and investing in new products and/or services which are in the introductory stage of the life cycle. In any case, the harvest strategy would include:

1. *Product.* The goal is to limit product investment and research and

EXHIBIT 6–17
Drop Strategy

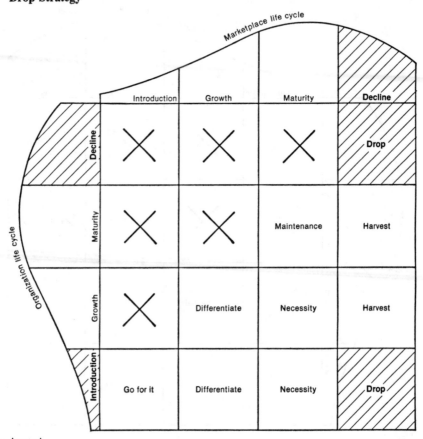

Legend
x = Position can not occur

development. Also, staff reduction may be necessary to keep costs down. Services may be more limited, such as reduced clinic hours. For example, in a pediatric practice, if one physician leaves, replacement may not be sought. Rather, expansion opportunities with other more promising specialties in an earlier life cycle phase may be considered.

2. *Price.* Tight cost controls must be maintained. And pricing should be profit-oriented, even though you may lose some market share. Avoid getting into competitive pricing wars.

3. *Promotion.* The basic promotion strategy is to again minimize expense in this phase. Avoid new promotion campaigns, but try to keep positive community relations through effective public relations strategies.

4. *Distribution*. The nature of a harvest strategy is to cut back, be efficient, maximize profit, and minimize new investment. Thus, the obvious distribution strategy is to shop expansion, eliminate marginal outlets or clinics, and drop marginal business.

Drop Strategy

This strategy is used when the market is in the decline stage and the organization life cycle is in the introduction stage *or* decline stage. In either case the same strategy applies. Clearly, if market conditions are in a decline stage, entry of another competitive product would be unwise—therefore the idea should be dropped. If both the OLC and MLC have moved to the decline stage, it would again be appropriate to drop the service, sell it, or merge with another entity. It is important to recognize that declining services tend to consume a disproportionate share of management time and financial resources.

■ Final Comments on the Match

The strategy action match provides the organization with direction for its marketing actions. Moreover, this approach follows the basis of the marketing approach outlined in Chapter 3. The match requires an external examination of the marketplace, as well as an internal assessment of the organization's position.

Successful position identification on each life cycle is determined by audits of the marketplace, competition, and organization. Throughout this chapter, data generated in staff work from Chapter 5 were required. As can be seen, the life cycle position, while not exact, must be reasonably accurate. Incorrect position placement can lead to strategies inconsistent with market demand.

After completion of the strategy action match, the organization can set its marketing objectives. Marketing objectives are specific target accomplishments which are consistent with the mission and the strategy action match. These objectives also form the basis for designing tactical actions. Whether or not marketing objectives are achieved will determine the extent to which the marketing plan is considered successful. Exhibit 6–18 provides examples of typical marketing objectives. Usually a marketing plan for a specific product or service will contain three to five specific marketing objectives.

Marketing objectives should be as precise as possible. Exhibit 6–19 provides guidelines which will help in developing specific marketing plans.

As Exhibit 6–19 indicates, typical objectives will include a measurable outcome such as units sold, market share, net income, or profit. Other objectives, such as image enhancement, may also be appropriate and can be measured with market research techniques. Objectives should also be developed within a time frame. Therefore, it is possible to measure results based on a specific time given to achieve the objective.

EXHIBIT 6-18
Sample Marketing Objectives

Objectives

1. Establish gross hospital revenue of $15 million in 198__.
2. Serve 110,000 (patient days/inpatient) in 198__.
3. Expand market share in Anytown, USA, from 18 percent total of inpatient hospital days to 22 percent by 198__.
4. Establish a gross margin across all product lines of 35 percent by 198__.
5. Establish a reputation among physicians and consumers as the number one, quality-rated heart surgery program in the state of Nevada by 198__.
6. Average 28 patients per physician, per practice day at an average billing of $30 per patient by 198__.
7. Harvest the service by the fourth quarter of 198__.
8. Become the market leader (in terms of market share) by 198__.

EXHIBIT 6-19
Guidelines for Setting Marketing Objectives

Marketing Objectives:
1. Should be measurable in dollars, time, and units.
2. Should be realistic.
3. Should be challenging.
4. Should be clear, concise, and understandable.
5. Should be consistent with one another.

In addition to the above guidelines, the following areas should be considered:
1. Profitability.
2. Cash flow.
3. Units sold.
4. Market share.
5. Image.
6. Quality.
7. Price.
8. Service.

Once the strategy action match has been completed, and appropriate marketing objectives developed, it is necessary to move on to the next step. This step involves developing those specific tactical actions which can be applied to meeting the objectives. The development of action strategies will be explored in the next chapter.

References

Ayal, Igal. "International Product Life Cycle: A Re-Assessment and Product Policy Implications." *Journal of Marketing* 45 (Fall 1981).

Bass, Frank M. "A New Product Growth Model for Consumer Durables." *Management Science* 15 (January 1969), pp. 215–27.

_____. "The Relationship Between Diffusion Rates, Experience Curves, and Demand Elasticities for Consumer Durable Technological Innovations." *Journal of Business* 53 (1980), pp. 551–67.

Buzzell, Robert D. "Competitive Behavior and Product Life Cycles." In *New Ideas for Successful Marketing,* eds. John Wright and Jac Goldstucker. Chicago: American Marketing Association, 1966.

Cardozo, Richard N. *Product Policy: Cases and Concepts.* Reading, Mass.: Addison-Wesley Publishing, 1979.

Catry, Bernard, and Chevalier Michel. "Market Share Strategy and the Product Life Cycle." *Journal of Marketing* 38 (October 1974), pp. 29–34.

Cox, William, Jr. "Product Life Cycles as Marketing Models," *Journal of Business* 40 (October, 1967), pp. 375–84.

Dhalla, Nariman, aad Sonya Yuspeh. "Forget the Product Life Cycle Concept." *Harvard Business Review* 54 (January/February 1976), pp. 102–12.

Dolan, Robert J., and Abel P. Jeuland. "Experience Curves and Dynamic Demand Models: Implications for Optimal Pricing Strategies." *Journal of Marketing* 45 (Winter 1981), pp. 52–73.

Enis, Ben M.; Raymond LaGarce; and Arthur E. Prell. "Extending the Product Life Cycle." *Business Horizons* 20 (June, 1977), pp. 46–56.

Harrell, Stephen G., and Elmer D. Taylor. "Modeling the Product Life Cycle for Consumer Durables." *Journal of Marketing* 45 (Fall 1981).

Harrigan, Kathryn Rudie. "Strategies for Declining Industries." *Journal of Business Strategy* 1 (Fall 1980), pp. 20–34.

Heeler, Roger M., and Thomas P. Hustad. "Problems in Predicting New Product Growth for Consumer Durables." *Management Science* 26 (October 1980), pp. 1007–1020.

Hofer, Charles W. "Toward a Contingency Theory of Business Strategy." *Academy of Management Journal* 18 (December 1975), pp. 784–810.

Levitt, Theodore. "Exploit the Product Life Cycle." *Harvard Business Review* 43 (November–December 1965), pp. 81–94.

Lillien, Gary L. "The Implictions of Diffusion Models for Accelerating the Diffusion of Innovation." *Technological Forecasting and Social Change* 17 (1980), pp. 339–351.

Mahajan, Vijay, and Eitan Muller. "Innovation Diffusion and New Product Growth Models in Marketing." *Journal of Marketing* 43 (Fall 1979), pp. 55–68.

Michael, George C. "Product Petrification: A New Stage in the Life Cycle Theory." *California Management Review* 9 (Fall 1971), pp. 88–91.

Midgley, David F. "Toward a Theory of the Product Life Cycle: Some Testable Propositions." *Journal of Marketing* 45 (Fall 1981).

Parsons, Leonard J. "The Product Life Cycle and Time-Varying Advertising Elasticities." *Journal of Marketing Research* 12 (November 1975), pp. 476–480.

Patel, Peter, and Michael Younger. "A Frame of Reference for Strategy Development." *Long Range Planning* 11 (April 1978), pp. 6–12.

Polli, Rolando, and Victor Cook. Validity of the Product life Cycle." *Journal of Business* 42 (October 1969), pp. 385–400.

Porter, Michael E. *Competitive Strategy*. New York: The Free Press, 1980.

Rink, David R., and John E. Swan. "Product Life Cycle Research: A Literature Review." *Journal of Business Research* 78 (September 1979), pp. 219–242.

Robinson, B., and C. Lakhani. "Dynamic Price Models for New Product Planning." *Management Science* 21 (June 1975), pp. 1113–22.

Thorelli, Hans B., and Stephen C. Burnett. "The Nature of Product Life Cycles for Industrial Goods Businesses." *Journal of Marketing* 45 (Fall 1981).

Tigert, Douglas, and Behrooz Farivar. "The Bass New Product Growth Model: A Sensitivity Analysis for a High Technology Product." *Journal of Marketing* 45 (Fall 1981).

Wasson, Chester R. *Product Management*. St. Charles, Ill.: Challenge Books, 1971.

Webster, Frederick E., Jr. "New Product Adoption in Industrial Markets: A Framework for Analysis." *Journal of Marketing* 33 (July 1969), pp. 35–39.

Wind, Yoram. *Product Policy: Concepts, Methods, and Strategy*. Reading, Mass.: Addison-Wesley Publishing, 1981.

Zaltman, Gerald, and Ronald Stiff. "Theories of Diffusion." In *Consumer Behavior: Theoretical Sources*, eds. Scott Ward and Thomas S. Robertson. Englewood Cliffs, N.J.: Prentice-Hall, 1972.

CHAPTER 7

DETERMINING MARKETING ACTIONS—STEP 4

Step 4: Determining Marketing Actions

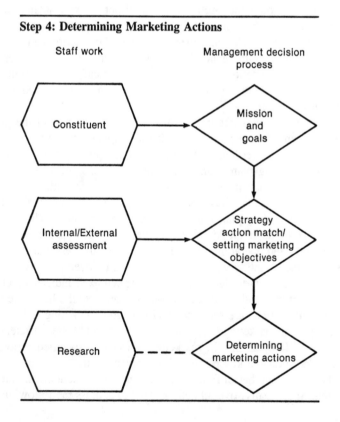

Step 4 is the process of translating marketing objectives into specific actions. This approach is based on the research of market wants and needs. Additional market research might also be used in Step 4 to forecast how successful the proposed action plan would be. Appendix B presents a review of alternative marketing research methodologies.

Continued coordination between the strategy action match and action plans is important. In Exhibit 6–10 several strategy options were outlined. These options are dependent upon the completion of a comprehensive analysis of the market, competition, internal analysis, internal organization, marketing review, and the strategy action match.

Frequently health care marketing managers put together marketing actions that are strategically weak. For example, an objective of increasing business, profitability, or the number of patients is often not followed through with a successful methodology for a competitive environment. An organization might be so good and successful that it is able to steal market share from a competitor. Little consideration is given to the possibility that the competitor may retaliate with protective countermeasures or by initiating intense, successful marketing actions of its own.

Therefore, it is important to establish strategically sound actions as discussed in the previous chapter. The objectives for these actions should be specific regarding outcome. Action must spell out in exact detail what must be done to achieve these marketing objectives and there must be detailed action developed for each major element of the plan. Action can be divided into two components—the general marketing action, such as the intention to establish a price-competitive product, and the tactical details outlining how that product will be competitive. This second component is called a *marketing implementation task*.

Development of marketing actions is the creative part of the process. The development and execution of marketing implementation tasks are more tedious activities. Nevertheless, both parts of the process are critical to the success of marketing plans. Once appropriate actions and tasks have been specified, the potential impact of these plans should be studied.

Finally, it is at this phase that marketing must act as a catalyst to help integrate the marketing plan into the overall business plan. The marketing staff should provide input to other members of the organization, such as those in finance and operations, to evaluate the effectiveness and "fit" of the proposed course of action within the organization's overall plans.

The sample market plan contained in Appendix C indicates that a reasonable amount of detail work is necessary to complete the life cycle match, determine what actions are required, and construct marketing tasks in order to accomplish the marketing objective. The plan should have sufficient detail regarding the life cycle match, marketing objectives, specified actions, and specific tasks to enable key personnel to implement it.

There are a number of functional elements of any action which must be considered. Specifically, overall actions need to address the following areas:

Product/service

Pricing

Distribution

Communications/promotion

Each of these elements will be discussed in detail.

■ Product/Service

The product or service is, to a great extent, the central element of the marketing mix. The life cycle has long been the foundation for decisions on product actions. There are several aspects of products/services about which the manager or group must make a decision. These decisions include selecting among possible new offerings, modifying existing services, choosing a branding strategy, and picking a program name. Each of these areas is discussed in this section.

Selecting among New Offerings

According to the life cycle concept, managers must recognize that decline may occur because of factors beyond their control. Therefore, a successful organization is always considering new service offerings. In Exhibit 7–1 a new service evaluation checklist is presented. This chart provides a score for each service offering to aid in the ranking of alternatives. The criteria provided on the checklist are not intended to be all-encompassing. Rather, each organization should specify the relevant criteria for alternative evaluation. And, where appropriate, add or delete criteria provided on the list. The value of the checklist is to provide a total picture in one of the most critical decision areas for any organization, the new service offering. This approach will also help in the selection of product alternatives, such as those shown in Exhibit 7–2.

Identifying product opportunities often requires creativity by key management personnel. In considering new program opportunities, the five questions outlined in Exhibit 7–3 may be helpful.

Modifying Existing Services

Often, as the market for a program or service matures, or more competitors enter the market, the need to modify the existing service offering arises. Program modifications are often accomplished in two ways.

Feature addition. One strategy to modify a program is by adding features to the existing offering. For example, part of an executive fitness program could now include a four-day residential program. This new feature would be conducted at a resort within a relatively easy drive of the hospital or clinic.

100

EXHIBIT 7–1
New Service Evaluation Checklist

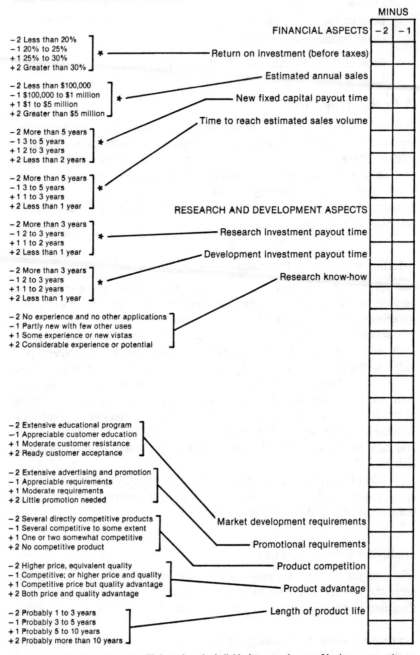

*The ratings for this aspect will depend on the individual company's type of business, accounting methods, and financial objective. The values shown above are estimated on the basis of various published information to bracket the averages for large chemical companies.

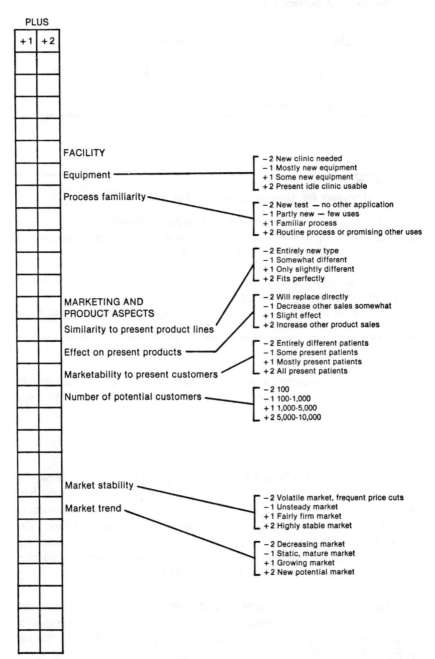

PLUS

+1	+2

FACILITY

Equipment ────────────────────────

- −2 New clinic needed
- −1 Mostly new equipment
- +1 Some new equipment
- +2 Present idle clinic usable

Process familiarity

- −2 New test — no other application
- −1 Partly new — few uses
- +1 Familiar process
- +2 Routine process or promising other uses

- −2 Entirely new type
- −1 Somewhat different
- +1 Only slightly different
- +2 Fits perfectly

**MARKETING AND
PRODUCT ASPECTS**

Similarity to present product lines

- −2 Will replace directly
- −1 Decrease other sales somewhat
- +1 Slight effect
- +2 Increase other product sales

Effect on present products ────────

- −2 Entirely different patients
- −1 Some present patients
- +1 Mostly present patients
- +2 All present patients

Marketability to present customers

Number of potential customers ────────

- −2 100
- −1 100-1,000
- +1 1,000-5,000
- +2 5,000-10,000

Market stability

- −2 Volatile market, frequent price cuts
- −1 Unsteady market
- +1 Fairly firm market
- +2 Highly stable market

Market trend

- −2 Decreasing market
- −1 Static, mature market
- +1 Growing market
- +2 New potential market

Source: John S. Harris, "New Product Profile Chart" *Chemical and Engineering News 39* (April 17, 1961) pp. 114–115. Reprinted with permission, Copyright 1982 American Chemical Society.

EXHIBIT 7−2
Examples of Service Innovations

1. Hospital-based retirement condominiums.
2. Portable CT-scanning offered to primary care physicians by radiologists.
3. First aid training programs for coaches and high school trainers.
4. Stress testing at tennis clubs and athletic facilities.
5. Opening a "hospi-tel."

EXHIBIT 7−3
Guiding Questions for Generating Service Innovations

1. Can this product substitute for another product? Example: surgi-center
2. Is it possible to combine this product or service with another to enhance the product line? Example: occupational health
3. Is it possible to adapt existing products or services into new products?
4. Is it possible to modify current products to become more competitive? Example: one-day OB package
5. Is it possible to magnify the product into a larger role than it has had in the past?

Quality shifting. A second strategy to modify a service is an actual quality change. As competition becomes more intense, the quality may be improved to seek differentiation.

The Branding Decision

The Johnston Clinic has been a multispecialty group for 20 years. Now, the organization has decided to get into the area of family practice in a suburb of their community where younger families have been establishing residence. What should this group be called? The Johnston Family Practice Clinic? The Johnston Clinic of Suburbia? Sound like a familiar problem? The branding strategy decision is important, and the health care manager should recognize the alternative trade-offs of each branding policy.

The blanket branding approach. With this strategy, an organization brings out every new product offering under one name. Think of the companies which follow this approach—Toro, Scott, Caterpillar, Medtronic, and the Humana Medfirst division.

The advantages of this strategy are obvious. The organization name carries over and reduces the cost of new service introduction. If the organization has a positive name, the consumer is more receptive to the introduction. The Johnston Clinic is a well-respected group in the community. Announcing an office in the suburban area may be seen as an extension of this well-known multispecialty group.

The blanket branding strategy, however, has its risks. A new service offering, not up to the high standards of the organization, may hurt the entire group. Therefore, the riskier the offering and the less time spent in research and development, the less attractive is the blanket branding approach.

Multibrand strategy. An alternative to the blanket brand strategy is the multibrand approach. The Johnston Clinic is merging with a group of family practitioners in the suburb. Some concerns exist about a couple of the physicians within this group. And, the Johnston Clinic recognizes that there is a significant percentage of the community which has always viewed the clinic as a high-priced group. The Johnston Clinic may decide to name the new group the "Suburbia Family Practice Clinic."

This strategy minimizes risk to the parent organization. Also, a multibrand approach can help attract a broad range of market segments. In using the "Suburbia" name, the physicians of the Johnston Clinic recognize that additional monies will have to be spent in introducing this "new" group to the community. However, the high-price image of the Johnston Clinic will not be carried over to this brand name.

Both branding approaches have their merits. Managers must consider the strategy and cost implications of each method.

Selecting the Program Name

The final product decision is the actual program name. Major corporations spend many dollars in selecting the "right name," yet the importance of this aspect has escaped many health care organizations. For example, with the strength of the name, Mayo Clinic, this organization could probably open family medicine clinics in most major markets in the United States and be assured of success.

The guidelines for name selection are simple. The name should be:

Meaningful. A program name should be relevant to the market for which it is developed. For example, Regional Oncology Programs means little to the community at large. The nonmedical person does not talk about oncology, but rather about cancer. Also, Ambulatory Care Centers sound like places in which ambulances are repaired.

Concise. Most good product names are short and crisp.

Easy to spell and pronounce. Otolaryngologists have recognized this concern by listing themselves in the Yellow Pages under "Ear, Nose, and

Throat." Many rheumatologists have provided alternative listings under "Arthritis." What is an endocrinologist?

Legal. Any service or product name should be free of legal ramifications.

The product/service decision is a challenging element of the marketing mix. Deciding which new service offering to develop, modifying existing services, choosing the appropriate branding strategy, and selecting the brand name are the key elements of service management.

■ Distribution

Distribution is another element of the marketing mix. This factor refers to the manner in which the service is delivered or offered to the customer or patient. In traditional industries, the channel of distribution refers to the linkages between the manufacturer, wholesaler, retailer, and consumer. Whereas this approach is considered the common path as a product moves from producer to buyer, channel variations exist. A similar analogy can be made in health care.

Exhibit 7–4 shows several distribution alternatives common to the health care setting. These can be characterized as direct or indirect. A direct channel exists when the service provider deals directly with the user. An example, is a primary care clinic which serves its immediate neighborhood. An indirect channel provides services with the assistance of an intermediary. This channel is illustrated by an orthopedic group which depends on referrals from primary care physicians. A hospital which provides services with the assistance of the medical staff is another indirect channel. A third form uses a sales force to sell the service to a buyer, such as a corporation, who may or may not be the direct user. Many hospital-based programs are beginning to sell through a sales force. In either direct or indirect channels, several decision areas exist.

Direct Channels

When direct distribution channels are used, the decisions focus on the following aspects:

Location. This decision aspect is possibly the most critical element for direct channels. *Where* should the facility be located? Often this decision has been made for the convenience of the practicing physicians. As competition for patients increases, however, location may be determined by the patients' preferences rather than by those of the professional staff.

Hours. The second decision aspect of distribution is *when* the service is to be available. Hours and days must meet the market's needs. For example, if

EXHIBIT 7–4
Distribution Alternatives

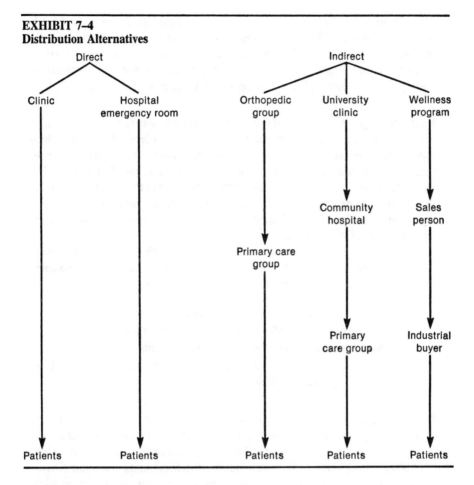

a group's patient base consists of families in which both husband and wife work, evening hours may be desirable.

Mode. The manner in which a service is distributed is a third aspect. This element entails *how* the service will be provided. Should all innoculations be provided by the physician at the primary care group? Or can a nurse provide this service? The mode by which a service is delivered can be altered for a competitive advantage in terms of price (as the latter example might provide) or in another dimension such as convenience, perceived quality, etc.

Indirect Channels

Each of the following decision areas pertains to indirect channels as well as direct channels. Yet in indirect channel settings, there are additional strategy concerns focusing on push/pull alternatives.

In an indirect channel, such as a tertiary hospital, patients can be admitted in two ways. The common method is to have patients referred to the hospital by the family physician. An alternative way to become an inpatient is for the patient himself to select the facility, such as a tertiary hospital or specialty clinic. Any indirect channel has two options, then, to attract users:

Push strategy. The push strategy is the traditional approach used by clinics and hospitals dependent on referrals. This approach centers on building loyalty among the members of the channel. Because of this loyalty, channel members will then push business to the specialty clinic or hospital. For example, through ongoing outreach efforts to physicians, the Fosston Cardiac Clinic has established a reputation of high-quality medicine. When primary care physicians face cardiac problems, they encourage (and direct) patients to the Fosston Clinic.

Successful implementation of a push strategy thus requires the development of loyalty from intermediate channel members. Common approaches to establishing this loyalty are to:

Provide special servicies (i.e., easy/quick scheduling) for doctors who regularly refer to your group or use your hospital.

Sponsor educational programs for channel members.

Offer direct incentives (office space in the attached medical building) to heavy physician admitters.

Pull strategy. An alternative to depending on the other channel members is to develop a preference for your facility among the ultimate users. For example, in many cities physicians may have privileges at several hospitals. Hospital X and Hospital Y both have modern obstetrical units. Hospital X tries to meet physicians' needs in a manner similar to its competitor. As an additional strategy, however, Hospital X attempts to pull patients into the hospital (around the physician). The hospital promotes its obstetrical service to consumers in the community. This promotion is done mainly by newspaper advertising. The objective of this approach is to have the patient *request* Hospital X when in the physician's office. In order for a pull strategy to work, the organization's quality of medical care, as well as its capabilities, must meet that of its competitors. Pull strategies are conducted mainly with the promotion element of the marketing mix.

■ Pricing

Some managers still believe that pricing does not apply to the health care industry. This view is not too surprising because of the traditional cost-based reimbursement system. However, third-party carriers who pay for the care

are developing competitive models, including HMOs, PPOs, and other payment schemes. As time goes on, price appears to be gaining strength as an important factor in the health care marketing environment. Physician-based insurance carriers, insurance carriers in general, the government, and other constituencies all have an interest in how health care services are being priced. In Chapter 1 some of the alternative reimbursement plans were reviewed. A common characteristic of all these plans is the emphasis on price competition. As reimbursement plans change, it will be increasingly appropriate to consider various pricing options.

Pricing strategies will differ, depending on goals and their direction. In general, costs determine the floor for pricing, and consumers set the ceiling. This allows for a variety of pricing actions which a hospital or clinic might consider. For example, listed below are several objectives which would result in various pricing actions:

1. Build traffic or market share.
2. Obtain short-run or long-run profits.
3. Obtain growth.
4. Stabilize the market.
5. Speed the exit of marginal competitors.
6. Discourage competitive entry.
7. Enhance image.
8. Develop product leadership.
9. Use price as an artificial determinant of quality.
10. Build traffic.

Factors that determine price include cost, competition, demand, and whether or not it is reimbursable. Depending on these factors, there are several different pricing actions that may be appropriate.

Skim Pricing

Skim pricing involves pricing at a high level. Buyers who are most interested in a service are less price sensitive and will find it acceptable to pay a higher price. This high price allows the organization to recover costs of project development. Moreover, a premium price can be used to develop a status position for the service in the consumer mind. Expensive cars, condominiums, some nursing homes, and consultants are examples of skim-pricing strategy. For example, a cosmetic surgery program may have a high price for status as well as for perceived quality implications. Who, for instance, would want to go to the "cheapest" cosmetic surgery program? Instead, buyers are likely to gravitate to the more expensive program which is perceived to be better. The use of a skim-pricing approach often encourages competitors to enter the market. A new competitor will seek to establish a new differential advantage based on a better price.

Penetration Pricing

Penetration pricing means pricing below the prevailing level in order to gain market entry or increase market share. Savin Copiers used this strategy to obtain a late entry into the copier market. This is the type of strategy PPOs are using. It is a method often used by organizations attempting to establish themselves within a market category. The Swedish Hospital decides to compete in the OB area with a low-cost, short-stay program. The prevailing community OB price is $2000. Swedish enters with a penetration price of $795 for 72 hours stay and a free steak dinner. Clearly, penetration pricing requires a good understanding of the organization's cost structure.

Elasticity Pricing

Elasticity pricing is used to take advantage of known or perceived price elasticity or inelasticity at a given point in time. For example, a parking space at a city hospital may be rented for $4 per space during the day shift hours and $1 per space during the evening hours. This pricing is based on demand elasticity.

Cost-Plus Pricing

Cost-plus pricing is the methodology which hospitals and clinics most often utilize. Reimbursement is generally made on this basis. This method can cause perception problems with consumers. For example, standard markups on items such as aspirin and chest X-rays are highly visible to consumers. Therefore standard markups on these items may be unwise. A better strategy would be to use variable pricing, which calls for shifting prices based on demand, customer expectation, and costs.

Numerous examples of other pricing strategies are also available. Hospitals and health care professionals are often somewhat limited in their use of pricing strategies. But, as there is more experimentation with nontraditional areas of health care, alternative pricing approaches will have to be used. Exhibit 7–5 illustrates various strategy-pricing examples.

EXHIBIT 7–5
Strategy-Pricing Examples

1. Package prices for husband/wife physical exams.
2. Providing patients with a discount for cash payment.
3. Prepayment pricing strategies for an OB program.
4. Industrial rates for companies that bring their accident victims to your hospital.
5. Family credit card programs.
6. Discounts (based on DRG code) to group buyers such as an industrial plant.

Exhibit 7–6 offers ideas on which pricing strategy to use, given various objectives and life cycle considerations. This chart indicates that a variety of pricing options is available under differing market conditions. It is apparent that, depending on the objective of the organization, pricing can be used as a tool to impact not only the financial performance of the company, but also the perceived quality and value of the service.

As hospitals and clinics become more competitive, pricing will become a more important tool. HMOs, PPOs, and others will continue to be price sensitive. However, different segments of the market will respond differently to price changes. Many buyers will be attracted to the higher-priced health care option, believing that high prices mean better service, better doctors, and better care. As a result, managers who consider raising or lowering prices must be sensitive to market reactions.

We can expect that health care institutions will begin to experiment more with pricing options beyond a cost-basis methodology. As a result, the marketing staff will begin to play a more important role, working with finance in the development of pricing strategies for health care organizations.

■ Promotion

Promotion has been the most visible aspect of marketing and of the most concern recently among health care professionals. Promotion consists of four elements:

Advertising.
Public relations.
Sales promotion.
Personal selling.

In the remainder of this book, public relations actions are not discussed because of the existing expertise of most health care professionals in this area. The other elements are discussed under the general headings of "advertising" and "sales."

■ Advertising

Advertising decisions revolve around two central issues—copy strategy and media selection. In both instances, the organization must have a defined target audience on which to focus its advertisements and a differential advantage attractive to the target audience. Unlike public relations pieces, the majority of all advertising copy is pretested among a sample of consumers representative of the target audience. There are several copy-testing alternatives.

EXHIBIT 7–6
Pricing Strategy Chart

Objective	Strategy	When Generally Used	Procedure	Advantages	Disadvantages
High short-term profit (without re-gard for long term).	Skim-the-cream of the market.	1. No comparable competitive products. 2. Drastically im-proved product or new product in-novation. 3. Large number of buyers. 4. Little danger of competitor entry due to high price, patent control, high R&D costs, high promotion costs, and/or raw material control. 5. Uncertain costs. 6. Short life cycle. 7. Inelastic demand.	Determine preliminary cus-tomer reaction. Charge premium price for product distinctiveness in the short run, without considering long run position. Some buyers will pay more be-cause of higher present value to them. Then, gra-dually reduce price to tap successive market levels - (i.e., skimming-the-cream of market that is relatively insensitive to price. Final-ly, tap more sensitive seg-ments).	1. Cushions against cost overruns. 2. Requires smaller in-vestment. 3. Provides funds quickly to cover new product promotions and initial development costs. 4. Limits demand until production is ready. 5. Suggests higher value in buyer's mind. 6. Emphasizes value rather than costs as a guide to pricing. 7. Allows initial feeling-out of demand before full-scale production.	1. Assumes that a market exists at high price. 2. Results in ill will by early buyers when price is reduced. 3. Attracts competi-tion. 4. Likely to under-estimate ability of competitors to copy products. 5. Discourages some buyers from trying the product (connotes high profits). 6. May cause long-run inefficiencies.

| Become established as efficient manufacturer at optimum volume before competitors get entrenched, without sacrificing long-term objectives (e.g., obtain satisfactory share of market). | Slide-down demand curve (version of skimming, without sacrificing long-term objectives). | 1. By established companies launching innovations.
2. Durable goods.
3. Slight barriers to entry by competition.
4. Medium life span. | Taps successive layers of demand at highest prices possible. Then slides down demand curve faster and further than forced to in view of potential competition. Rate of price change is slow enough to add significant volume at each successive price level but fast enough to prevent large competitor from becoming established on a low-cost volume basis. | 1. Emphasizes value rather than cost as a guide to pricing.
2. Provides rapid return on investment.
3. Provides slight cushion against cost overruns. | 1. Requires broad knowledge of competitive product developments.
2. Requires much documented experience.
3. Results in ill will by early buyers when price is reduced.
4. Discourages some buyers from buying at initial high price. |
| Encourage others to produce and promote the product to stimulate primary demand. | Competitive-at-the-market price. | 1. Several comparable products.
2. Growing market.
3. Medium-to-long product life span.
4. Known costs. | Start with final price and work back to cost. Use customer surveys and studies of competitors' prices to approximate final price; deduct selling margins; adjust product and production and selling methods to sell at this price and still make necessary profit margins. | 1. Requires less analysis and research.
2. Existing market requires less promotion efforts.
3. Causes no ill will by early buyers since price will not be lowered soon. | 1. Limited flexibility.
2. Limited cushion for error.
3. Slower recovery of investment.
4. Must rely on other differentiating tools. |

(continued)

EXHIBIT 7 – 6 (continued)

Objective	Strategy	When Generally Used	Procedure	Advantages	Disadvantages
Stimulate market growth and capture and hold a satisfactory market share at a profit through low prices. Become strongly entrenched to generate profits over a long period.	Market penetration.	1. Long product life span. 2. Mass market. 3. Easy market entry. 4. Demand is highly sensitive to price. 5. Unit costs of production and distribution decrease rapidly as quantity of output increases. 6. Newer product. 7. No "elite" market willing to pay premium for newest and best.	Charge low prices to create a mass market resulting in cost advantages derived from larger volume. Look at lower end of demand curve to set price low enough to attract a large customer base. Also review past and competitor prices.	1. Discourages actual and potential competitor inroads because of apparent low profit margins. 2. Emphasizes value more than cost in pricing. 3. Allows maximum exposure and penetration in minimum time. 4. May maximize long-term profits if competition is minimized.	1. Assumes volume is always responsive to price reductions, which isn't always true. 2. Relies somewhat on glamour and psychological pricing which doesn't always work. 3. May create more business than production capacity available. 4. Requires significant investment. 5. Small errors often result in large losses.

(continued)

| Keep competitors out of market or eliminate existing ones. | Preemptive extinction. | 1. Used more often in consumer markets.
2. Manufacturers may use this approach on one or two products, with other prices meeting or higher than those of competitors. | Price at low levels so that market is unattractive to possible competitors. Set price as close as possible to total unit cost. As increased volume allows lower cost, pass advantage to buyers via lower price. If costs decline rapidly with increases in volume, can start price below cost. (Can use price approaching variable costs.) | 1. Discourages potential competitors because of apparent low profit margins.
2. Limits competitive activity and expensive requirements to meet them. | 1. Must offer other policies which permit lower price (limited credit, delivery, or promotions).
2. Small errors can result in large losses.
3. Long-term payback period. |

Source: Reprinted from Cochrane Chase and Kenneth Barasch, *Marketing Problem Solver* (Radnor, Pa.: Chilton), with permission of the publisher, © 1977, pp. 190-91.

Copy Testing

Copy testing occurs at two stages of the advertising process. *Pretesting* is conducted before the advertisement is placed in the media. Tests at this stage are made to determine which alternative advertising copy strategies should be used, the interest/attention-getting power of an advertisement or the meaning of the advertisement.

Copy format testing. Often it is desirable to develop more than one advertisement to consider. For example, the Merrimack Hospital has developed a pain clinic. The decision has been made to advertise the program in the newspaper. Two alternative ads are developed to tell the market about this program. One advertisement shows a person with one hand to his forehead and eyeglasses in the other hand. The person appears to be suffering from migraine. The second copy layout contains no picture, but a bold print definition of the word pain. Before these ads are run, they are shown to a group of people who are similar to the target audience for the program. Consumers are then asked to rate the advertisements in terms of which they prefer, which is of most interest to them, and which one best communicates the value of the hospital program. According to the market-based approach, it is the *intended* audience who should decide which of the alternative advertisements to run.

Readability and understandability. Before any advertisement is placed in the media, pretesting should be conducted to insure that it is understood by the market in the same way it was intended by the organization. This step is especially important in dealing with the two major market segments for most health care organizations—consumers and physicians.

Because of the technical vocabulary dominant in health care, interpretability is a central pretesting concern with consumers. The Wilkus Multispecialty Clinic advertises the addition of a new group member who specializes in endocrinology. An announcement is positioned in the local community paper. Good exposure, but the majority of consumers do not understand what or who has been added. The value of this announcement to consumers is thus lost.

In pretesting an advertisement for physicians, the purpose is less for comprehension and more for intention. That is, the sensitivity of advertising requires that physicians interpret the message as intended. A radio advertisement lead-in, designed solely to attract attention, may be seen as unprofessional by members of the medical staff.

Posttesting. This evaluation is conducted after the advertisement has been run in the appropriate media. Common posttesting procedures focus on *recall* or *recognition*. Recognition tests attempt to determine whether the target audience remembers seeing the advertisement. For example, a sample of consumers is shown the Wilkus Clinic ad and asked whether they remember seeing the endocrinologist announcement. An alternative is to assess the recall of an advertisement. For example, the Merrimack Hospital decided to run its Pain Clinic ad with the picture version in the local newspaper. A random sample of consumers is called two days after the ad runs. Consumers are first asked whether they read the local paper. They are then asked whether they *recall* any health care advertisements during the past week. If yes, *what* was the advertisement.

Other tests of advertising are more directly related to measures of effectiveness. These approaches are discussed in greater detail in a later section.

Media Selection

Related to the copy strategy decision is the selection of media. The vast majority of clinics and hospitals make media decisions on a local basis. Yet because of technological advances, media once out of reach of most local advertisers are now part of any good media plan. Cable television, local spot time, and zip code (and metro) editions of national magazines allow a broader media plan.

Following is a review of the major considerations with each medium.

Newspapers. The advantage of newspapers is coverage. As many clinics and hospitals have found, a vast majority of adults report reading a newspaper at least once in the course of any week. Moreover, newspapers allow for quick competitive response. If the competing clinic runs a newspaper ad on Monday, the other clinic can retaliate with very short lead time through the newspaper. Advertising space is available on relatively short notice.

The major disadvantage with newspapers is a lack of selectivity. Although many large papers have added zip code editions, this selectivity is less common outside major metropolitan areas. Consequently, when the Rockville Hospital runs an advertisement for its executive fitness program, many nonexecutives will see it. If the program is not intended for this audience, the hospital has paid for wasted coverage.

Magazines. Magazines have become a popular medium in the United States. The proliferation of special interest magazines allows the potential advertiser to reach a specific target audience. The HMO may run an advertisement in its area's regional edition of *Prevention* magazine. People who read this publication are concerned with health and wellness. An ad focusing on the "health maintenance" position of the organization might have special appeal. *Runner's World* might be a suitable outlet for a large clinic or hospital which wants to establish a nationally known sports medicine program.

The major disadvantage of magazines may pertain to cost. Publication costs can be high. However, as numerous magazines develop regional/metro editions of their publications, costs become more affordable for the hospital or group practice.

Direct mail. Of all media available to health care organizations, direct mail provides maximum selectivity. Direct mail houses can provide assistance in mailing communications to defined target audiences. For example, the Merrimack Hospital has decided to focus its pain clinic on individuals of 60 years of age or older who have arthritis. With the assistance of a direct mail house, a brochure on the pain program can be sent to that specific group in the desired market area.

The major obstacle to direct mail is its classification as junk mail. The volume of unsolicited mail received is often overwhelming. However, well-designed, professional pieces about an issue of importance to the target audience can generate response.

Radio. Many clinics and hospitals have turned to radio to generate awareness. The vast number of radio stations means that some selectivity with regard to the target audience is possible. A teenage drug counseling program at Community Hospital is advertised on the local station which plays rock music. Radio is a relatively low-cost vehicle, and many stations will help in writing and producing the advertisement.

The major weakness of radio is the ease with which the message can be tuned out. Long advertisements are not possible, and even with a short spot, the individual can tune out by hitting a preset button to switch stations.

Television. Although five years ago few health care managers would have thought of television for anything but public service announcements, more organizations have turned to this medium. The advantage is the potential for sight and sound. Television can reach a large number of people, but also has some selectivity.

The major disadvantage for most organizations is cost. Television commercials are expensive to produce. And the cost of placement is often high. While low-cost space is available at most local stations, the time slots often reach an audience which may not match the desired target group. Inexpensive time can be purchased from most television stations during the late, late show. The key question is "who's watching?" This time slot may be perfect for the clinic's sleep program, but is of little value for the fitness program.

Outdoor advertising. Billboards have gained increasing popularity with many health care organizations. This medium is very effective for awareness and as a supplementary effort to other advertising. However, using billboards as the only medium in an advertising campaign is not sufficient.

A major disadvantage of outdoor advertising is that the message must be short and simple. Also, little selectivity of the people who view the advertisement is possible. Moreover, in some cities obtaining billboard space in the desired location is difficult.

Exhibit 7–7 presents a summary of the media along selected decision criteria. Appropriate media selection requires a knowledge of the viewership, readership, and even the travel patterns of the target audience.

Measuring effectiveness and setting objectives are some of the more difficult aspects of advertising. While it may be desirable to advertise and see an increase in outpatient visits to the ambulatory care center of 10 percent during the month of the campaign, it's not always so easy. Competitive actions and the lag effect of advertising can influence the outcome of an ad campaign. Advertising campaigns need a set of measurable objectives. Some precampaign assessment of the goals is also needed. Logical objectives for an advertising campaign might include:

> To increase name recognition of the Wallace Clinic from 10 percent to 25 percent within nine months, among people who have moved into the community within the past six months.
>
> To have 35 percent of the consumers in zip codes contingent to the hospital express a preference for our hospital's ER service in the next two months.
>
> To generate 15 inquiries a month from eligible corporations about our occupational health program.

Again, a specific, measurable objective must be provided in order to evaluate whether or not the advertising works. Setting advertising objectives should be conducted in light of the "hierarchy of effects" which a potential buyer goes through. These steps are:

Awareness. The potential buyer is aware that the product/service exists in the market.

Interest. The potential buyer is aware of the concept and wants more information regarding the offering.

Evaluation. The customer attempts to evaluate the relative benefits of one offering to another.

Trial. The customer is interested in trying the service on a limited scale.

Adoption. The customer decides to utilize the service on a regular basis.

It is difficult to set advertising objectives around the focus of adoption or utilization. The primary reason is that several factors may affect utilization, such as whether your plan is offered by the potential patient's company,

EXHIBIT 7-7
Selection Trade-offs with Alternative Media

	Cost of Placement	Selectivity	Message Quality	Lead Time
Newspapers	Relatively expensive.	Little selectivity except in major metro areas. By zip code or region.	Poor photo reproduction. Person can spend time with message.	Easy to obtain space with short notice.
Magazines	Relatively expensive.	Great selectivity by lifestyle, interest. Reasonably good selectivity by area (particularly metro).	Excellent photo reproduction. Person can spend time with message.	Often requires contracting for space with a month or more prior notice.
Direct mail	Relatively inexpensive.	Excellent selectivity on criteria required by organization.	Excellent as a function of dollars spent in printing.	Little required except to produce mail piece.
Radio	Inexpensive.	Reasonable selectivity.	Must be short, simple. Difficult to hold attention.	Little advance notice required to run a commercial.
Television	Expensive.	Reasonable—a function of time of day and show selected.	Excellent for sight and sound. Relatively short messages required. Hard to hold attention.	Often requires substantial lead time with station for time.
Outdoor	Relatively inexpensive.	Little selectivity except by location of billboard.	Requires short, simple message.	Space availability often requires long lead time.

EXHIBIT 7-8
Possible Hierarchy Objectives

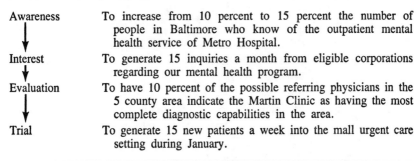

Awareness	To increase from 10 percent to 15 percent the number of people in Baltimore who know of the outpatient mental health service of Metro Hospital.
Interest	To generate 15 inquiries a month from eligible corporations regarding our mental health program.
Evaluation	To have 10 percent of the possible referring physicians in the 5 county area indicate the Martin Clinic as having the most complete diagnostic capabilities in the area.
Trial	To generate 15 new patients a week into the mall urgent care setting during January.

the existing medical need of the patient, or the referral problem faced by the physician. Particularly in health care, with the episodic nature of medical problems, an organization can never be sure when exposure to an advertisement may lead to eventual utilization.

Recognizing that a person's medical need may lag behind awareness of an advertisement for a group's service does not imply that advertising effects are unmeasurable. Rather, the objective by which advertising effectiveness can be evaluated must be set at levels before adoption or utilization. Exhibit 7-8 shows some possible objectives at earlier levels of the hierarchy. The objectives listed in the exhibit provide for a possible measure of advertising which might be readily observable. As one moves down the hierarchy, however, more active behavior (such as trial) is required.

Without measurable objectives, an organization can never be sure whether advertising is working or not. Advertising budgets become hard to justify as fear builds up that advertising cannot be reduced. Before any expenditures are made, objectives must be established.

Setting the Budget

Early concerns over advertising often pertained to issues of reimbursement. Advertising is not a reimbursable expense. Yet each year more health care organizations are realizing it is an important way to compete. A recent study indicated most hospitals project an ever-increasing budget for advertising.[1] Setting an exact budget amount is difficult, but there are several common approaches.

All you can afford. This approach for determining the advertising budget is common to many professional organizations. In developing the operating budget for the coming fiscal year, dollars are allocated to personnel, oper-

---

[1] Eric Berkowitz, Steven Hillestad and Pamela Effertz, "The Future of Advertising: A Hospital Perspective," *Journal of Health Care Marketing* 2, no. 3 (Summer 1982), p. 39.

EXHIBIT 7 – 9
Advertising and Promotion Budget as
a Percentage of Total Sales

	Percent
Optical instruments	3.6
Medical instruments	3.1
Wholesale drugs	1.1
Restaurants	2.9
Ethical drugs	7.8
Grocery store chains	1.1

Source: *Sales and Marketing Management,*
February 22, 1982, p. 129.

---

ations, capital improvements, new equipment purchases, and the like. After all critical categories receive their allocated dollars, additional monies still remain. The clinic financial committee decides to use this to try advertising.

Certainly the financial viability of the organization must be a constraint in advertising. No banker has been found who will lend money for a group practice's advertising campaign. Yet the health care organization that follows this approach spends the available dollars on advertising just because they think they should be advertising. However, specific objectives have not been created to direct the campaign. This approach lacks logic.

Advertising as a percent of revenue. A second common budgeting strategy is allocating to advertising a percent of the group or hospital's revenue. Exhibit 7–9 shows some existing percentages for various industries. Again, this approach has some value in that advertising is tied to the financial performance of the organization. Of all budgeting methods, however, this approach may be the weakest. With this method, the hospital's revenue causes advertising, rather than advertising resulting in revenue. With this approach, an organization may reduce its advertising expenditures at the time the greatest investment is needed, when demand is down. Likewise, increasing revenue will lead to a greater advertising budget, although this new level of expenditure may not be warranted.

Competitive parity. As more health care organizations begin to advertise, competitive parity is becoming the budgeting model. The Mentor Clinic has observed the Austin Clinic's weekly newspaper advertising. As a countermeasure, the Mentor Clinic begins newspaper advertising.

When a major competitor advertises, it forces the organization to consider a retaliatory strategy. Yet spending advertising dollars at the same level as the competitor assumes similar organizational objectives. Moreover, the Mentor Clinic assumes the Austin Clinic knows what it is doing and that the strategy is correct. These assumptions are often tenuous.

Objective and task. There are components of each of the following budgeting methods which are important in any advertising allocation. Affordability, revenue, and competition must all be assessed. Yet the overriding weakness of each method is the lack of objectives. As noted in the preceding pages, the effectiveness of advertising can only be determined through prespecified objectives. These same objectives should guide the budget determination. Recall the awareness objective in Exhibit 7–8: "To increase from 10 percent to 15 percent the number of people in Baltimore who know of the outpatient mental health service of Metro Hospital."

Once the objective is set, the organization must determine how to meet this objective. How much media exposure is needed in newspapers, radio, television, etc. The tasks to meet the exposure are outlined. For example:

Tasks

Three insertions (¼ page) in the Baltimore Sun.

Four 20-second slots on the late news, Channel 5.

The costs to undertake these tasks are then calculated. This amount determines the budget.

It is also at this point that the previous factors of affordability, competition, and revenue enter. After determining the amount the organization has available for advertising, it may be found that the objectives cannot be financially supported. This discovery may lead to a readjustment of the objective or a search for more efficient media. Or, the budgeted amount may be well below competitive levels. This finding may require a more critical evaluation of the tasks and likelihood of success.

Of all methods, this final aproach requires the most planning. Yet the advantage overcomes this additional investment in management time. An objective-driven budget for advertising, based on accountable performance standards, is created. Advertising is an expensive and essential part of promotional strategy. Health care organizations need to plan this activity as carefully as they do the establishment of a new medical service.

■ Sales

While the authors were among the first to suggest the use of sales strategies years ago, personal selling is an area not used to a great extent by hospitals or clinics.[2] In fact, the effectiveness of a sales force has been underestimated by most health care organizations. To a great extent, this lack of use may be attributed to a professional concern about mixing "selling" and medicine. Yet the value of a sales staff can take many forms in addition to selling.

---

[2]Sales strategies were discussed before the American College of Hospital Administrators (ACHA) Congress in 1980 and 1979. Also, sales strategies were reviewed in the American Academy of Medical Directors Annual meeting, 1979.

Information

The more technical or complicated the service, the more valuable is a sales staff. Many of the programs offered by hospitals and clinics are probably better communicated to the market by a salesperson than by an advertisement. Consider the occupational health programs established by many clinics. The common strategy is to run an advertisement in the local business publication read by company executives. Because the decision to utilize a particular occupational health program is complicated and may be made by several management personnel, a personal sales strategy might be more effective. The clinic could establish a small sales force to call on local companies. The early sales calls would be to gain knowledge about the account. Who is involved in the health care plan decision? What are the occupational health needs of the company? What health care sources are presently used by the organization? After proper account knowledge, a more effective presentation of the clinic's own occupational health services could be made.

Relationship Maintenance

A valuable role of a sales staff is in maintaining relationships as much as in selling. This purpose is particularly relevant for hospitals which depend upon physician loyalty and clinics dependent on referrals from physicians and other individuals (such as probation officers, social workers, and employee assistance personnel). In fulfilling this function, the role of the salesperson is to ensure that the physician's needs are being met by the hospital and its staff. If salespeople uncover problems or areas of dissatisfaction, they can be the links to the administrator or program director. Moreover, the salesperson can act as a conduit of new information regarding the clinic's programs or changes.

Listed below are several markets on which a sales force might call. Each would be appropriate for specific programs, although the information-maintenance-sales purpose may vary. For example, a sales force could call on:

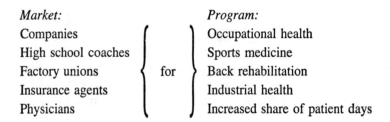

Market:		Program:
Companies		Occupational health
High school coaches		Sports medicine
Factory unions	for	Back rehabilitation
Insurance agents		Industrial health
Physicians		Increased share of patient days

In calling on any market, the sales force can fulfill one or several roles. In addition to those previously reviewed. Establishment of a personal selling function can be helpful for:

Actual sales. The basic purpose of any salesperson is to get utilization or close the sales. A hospital sales force for industrial medicine may be used to sign contracts with companies. A PPO sales force is used to sign doctors to the plan.

Clarification. A second important role of any sales force is for clarification. Salespeople can provide an explanation and evaluation of the clinic's new outpatient chemical dependency program.

Missionary. An important role of the sales force is missionary activity. In this role, the salesperson deals with the referral physician or company contact person. The goal is to help that individual's practice or business by the service provided by the hospital. The salesperson builds goodwill for the clinic as well as a sense of obligation with the primary care physician.

Satisfaction monitoring. In this final role, the salesperson monitors user satisfaction level. A salesperson regularly calls on physicians to see that the physicians' needs are being met. The salesperson can be the conduit for any complaints to the administration, before the physician begins to shift patients to another facility. Or, the company benefit officer is periodically called on to ensure that employee records provided by the HMO meet the company's cost review needs.

Many roles can be played by the salespeople, once it has been decided that they are necessary. There are two key areas of concern related to setting up the sales force. These are, the size of the sales force and the method of compensation.

The size of the sales force. There are several alternative methods for determining sales force size. Conceptually, the most appealing, as well as the easiest to implement, is the *work-load method*.

Work-load method. This is based on the work load each salesperson can handle. By measuring the load and dividing it into the total effort necessary to cover the entire market, the required number of salespeople is determined. This method, sometimes termed a *buildup approach,* consists of the following steps:

1. *Establish total time available per salesperson.* Suppose that the sales job requires working an eight-hour day, five days a week, calling on potential industrial accounts for an occupational health program. Eliminating four weeks for vacation, holidays, illness, and other emergencies leaves 48 working weeks in a year. The total number of hours per year a salesperson will work, on the average, will then be 1920 (40 hours per week $\times$ 48 weeks).

2. *Apportion salesperson's time to all required tasks.* A salesperson's time must be divided among many different tasks. For this example, the tasks can be grouped into selling, traveling, and nonselling categories. If territories are being established for the first time, the manager's estimates are often used to apportion time to these tasks. When already-established territories are being reviewed, the apportionment might be based on the salesperson's reports or time studies. Suppose the following breakdown of time was established for an average salesperson and applied to the total hours available:

Selling	40%	768 hours
Traveling	30%	576 hours
Nonselling	30%	576 hours
Total	100%	1920 hours

3. *Classify customers according to selling effort required.* Next the firm's present and potential customers must be classified in terms of selling effort required. Customers are usually grouped into sales volume categories, although any basis for grouping can be used as long as it distinguishes accounts according to differences needed in selling effort. For our occupational health program, we will group them by the number of employees in the firm. This can be a tedious task for a firm with many customers and prospects.

To continue the example, assume that the number of customers (both present and potential) classified by number of employees is as follows:

Group 1—Large	10 accounts
Group 2—Medium	25 accounts
Group 3—Small	100 accounts

4. *Specify length and frequency of call for each category.* The manager might use experimental evidence, his or her own judgment, or opinions of the sales force to determine how much time should be spent with an account in each group and how often each account should be visited. Potential as well as present customers must be included in this step, or else the final number of salespersons will not be large enough to allow cultivation of potential accounts.

To facilitate our example, suppose that present and potential customers are to be treated equally. The manager might then determine the following call frequencies and call lengths as ideal:

Group 1	24 calls per year × 45 minutes per call =	18 hours per year
Group 2	12 calls per year × 30 minutes per call =	6 hours per year
Group 3	4 calls per year × 30 minutes per call =	2 hours per year

Total time needed to cover all accounts would then be:

Group 1	10 accounts at 18 hours	= 180 hours
Group 2	25 accounts at 6 hours	= 130 hours
Group 3	100 accounts at 2 hours	= 200 hours
Total		510 hours

5. *Calculate number of salespersons needed.* Each salesperson has 768 hours available on the average for selling. Total selling time needed to cover present and potential accounts is 510 hours. By dividing 510 by 768, the result is approximately a .7 FTE for sales on industrial accounts.

The work-load method is easy to understand and carry out, and companies have used it with satisfying results.

The method of compensation. The second decision area is compensation. There are several elements to any compensation plan. They are:

Salary.

Commission.

Bonus.

Expense payments.

Fringe benefits.

Commission is a complicated element. The several components to consider are shown in Exhibit 7–10. Likewise, expense items can also vary.

EXHIBIT 7–10
Components to Compensation

Bases for Commission Payments
1. Dollar or unit sales volume (gross or net).
2. Gross margin, contribution to profit.
3. Activities or efforts.
4. Quotas (which may include above bases).

Rates of Commission
1. Fixed, progressive, regressive.
2. Gross versus net.
3. Constant versus variable with regard to:
   a. Products.
   b. Customers.
   c. Territories.
   d. Order sizes.
   e. Profit margins.
   f. New versus repeat business.

Starting Points for Commission Payments
1. Zero sales, profits or activities.
2. Some percentage of quota.
3. Break-even level of sales volume.

EXHIBIT 7 – 11
Common Sales Expense Items

80 Percent or More Firms Allow:

Meals: breakfast, lunch, dinner.
Taxis or other local transportation.
Room.
Railroad transportation.
Gratuities (all occasions).

50 Percent to 80 Percent of Firms Allow:

Valet, laundry while away from home.
Charges for excess baggage.
Restaurant entertainment.
Postage, telephone, telegrams to home.

20 Percent to 50 Percent of Firms Allow:

Cocktails.
Office supplies and equipment while away from home.
Travel insurance.
Night clubs.
Sporting events.
Theater.
Theft, loss, or damage to personal effects.

Source: Reprinted by permission of the publisher from Research Study no. 82, "Expense Account Control," by John N. Taussig, © 1967 by the American Management Association, Inc. All rights reserved.

Exhibit 7–11 shows expense items which are commonly reimbursed by companies.

The Advertising/Sales Trade-off

A major issue facing many managers is the balance between personal selling and advertising. No correct formula exists to solve this problem. Rather, it is important to recognize the contribution of each element in a proper promotional program. First, consider the nature of the purchase or utilization decision. When a doctor decides to send a patient to a referral center, there are three components to the decision. First is prepurchase. This stage is the deliberation the physician goes through before actually deciding on the referral center. Second is the purchase or, in this case, actual decision stage. The third phase is postpurchase. At this point the physician may review his decision to examine whether the right selection was made. Advertising and personal selling have different levels of effectiveness at each stage.

As shown in Exhibit 7–12 advertising assumes greater importance in the prepurchase stage. Advertising may consist of brochures distributed by the referral center to primary care providers, or it may be regional advertisements by an HMO in the Wall Street Journal. The purpose of a mass information approach (advertising) is to make as many prospective buyers or

---

EXHIBIT 7–12
Advertising/Sales Impact

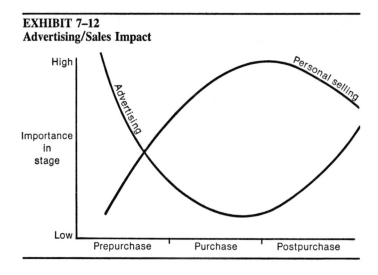

users aware of the service as possible. In the second stage, personal selling assumes greater importance. It is the rare advertisement which has ever closed a sale. To do this, the personal interaction between buyer and seller must occur. In the example of a primary care physician's referral, consider this possibility. There is a physician in the region who has never sent a patient to the Holt Orthopedic Group. Over the past years, however, Holt has undertaken extensive information awareness regarding their services. After a couple of preliminary calls on this primary care physician, the Holt representative (i.e., salesperson) asks the physician to try the group for her next orthopedic case (i.e., purchase). The salesperson is needed to bring closure. After the decision stage, note in Exhibit 7–12 that advertising is still important and so is personal selling. Often after making a decision when competing alternatives exist, a person questions the correctness of his actions. Advertising often serves to reduce the postdecision anxiety. The physician sees another advertisement or brochure for the group and feels at ease about the decision. Even better than advertising, however, is postpurchase personal contact. The more personal the contact with the buyer after the sales transaction, the more satisfied the buyer tends to be. In this example, the Holt representative returns to the referring physician to ensure documentation on the case was received, the patient's experience was positive, and that no other problem with this referral was encountered. This is also a good time to ask for increased loyalty. In deciding on the proper balance of advertising and sales, the organization must consider the feelings of the buyer as carefully as it does its own goals and objectives.

There are situations, however, when advertising should receive more attention than sales and vice versa. Exhibit 7–13 indicates some of the dimensions by which this trade off can be made. Each criterion is reviewed as described on p. 128.

EXHIBIT 7 – 13
Considerations in Using Sales People Versus Advertising

	More Emphasis on	
	Sales if:	*Advertising if*
Degree of technical sophistication	High	Low
Number of potential customers	Few	Many
Marketing strategy	Push	Pull
Composition of buyer decision-making unit	Complex	Simple
Ancillary services	Many	Few
Degree of risk	Great	Little

Degree of technical sophistication. The more technically complex the service being sold, the greater the need for personal sales. A salesperson can play a valuable role in explaining or communicating the benefits to the buyer, especially when these benefits may not be readily observable.

Number of potential customers. The more customers or potential buyers existing in the market, the greater the role of advertising. The cost per contact of advertising drops dramatically with more buyers, while with personal selling it increases. No hospital could have a personal sales force explain the value of its obstetrics service to potential patients. Yet a sales force calling on social workers in the community for the hospital-based mental health program may be feasible.

Marketing strategy. The nature of the organization's strategy dictates the relative emphasis on advertising or personal selling. As explained earlier, a pull strategy requires advertising. Salespeople are a prerequisite to a push strategy for working with the intermediates in the channel.

Composition of buyer decision-making unit. The more people involved in the decision to use a service, the greater the need for personal sales. Multiple decision makers often have different criteria regarding their evaluation of the service. A salesperson is valuable for explaining the program to each decision maker. This multiple explanation would be difficult to accomplish with any advertisement.

Ancillary services. This dimension refers to any postsales service that might be required. For example, the company may expect updates on employee utilization of the industrial medicine program. The referral physician expects documentation on any cases sent to the tertiary facility. In these instances, personal selling helps to provide the follow-ups discussed earlier. The salesperson is actually part of the "program" purchased by the buyer.

Degree of risk. The more risk the buyer sees in using a program, the more important are personal sales. This risk can be physical or financial. For example, a hospital-based, one-day surgery program may have orientation sessions for prospective users. At these sessions, a hospital salesperson can explain the concept and safeguards. Although the physician has suggested that one-day surgery is the way to do the procedure, a patient may view surgery as serious and not a one-day affair. The hospital sales program may be necessary to get patient compliance. Or else the patient may seek another physician who will comply with an inpatient request, but not at your hospital.

Advertising and personal selling are both important components for effective promotion. Health care organizations must realize that both elements have strong impact on the market at varying stages of the buying process.

Checklist for Chapter 7

1. Do specific tactics selected from the marketing mix match the life cycle strategy?
2. Are tactics realistic?
3. Are tactics specific?
4. Are you doing enough to make sure your goals are achieved?
5.. Have you considered the full range of marketing mix elements (product, price, promotion, distribution) in developing your strategy?

References

Advertising/Promotion:

DeLozier, M. Wayne. *The Marketing Communication Process.* New York: McGraw-Hill, 1976.

Engel, James F.; Martin R. Washaw; and Thomas C. Kinnean. *Promotional Strategy.* Homewood, Ill.: Richard D. Irwin, 1983.

McNiven, M. "Plan for More Productive Advertising." *Harvard Business Review,* March–April 1980.

Wolfe, Harry Dean; James K. Brown; Stephen H. Greenberg; and C. Clark Thompson. *Pretesting Advertising.* National Industrial Conference Board, Study #109, 1963.

Distribution:

Stern, Louis W., and Adel I. El-Ansaly. *Marketing Channels.* 2d ed. Englewood Cliffs, N.J.: Prentice-Hall, 1982.

Weigland, Robert. "Fit Products and Channels to Your Markets." *Harvard Business Review,* January–February 1977.

Pricing:

Dean, Joel. "Pricing Policies for New Products." *Harvard Business Review* 54 (November–December 1976), pp. 141–53.

Monroe, Kent B. *Pricing: Making Profitable Decisions.* New York: McGraw-Hill, 1979.

Oxenfeldt, Alfred R. *Pricing Strategies.* New York: American Management Association, 1975.

_____. "Product Line Pricing." *Harvard Business Review,* 44 (July–August 1966), pp. 137–44.

Shapiro, Benson P. "The Psychology of Pricing." *Harvard Business Review,* 46 (July–August 1968.) pp. 14–25, 160.

Product:

Buzzell, Robert D.; Bradley T. Gale; and R. G. M. Sultan. "Market Share—A Key to Profitability." *Harvard Business Review,* 53 (January–February 1975), pp. 97–106.

Cardozo, Richard N. *Product Policy: Cases and Concepts.* Reading, Mass.: Addison-Wesley Publishing, 1979.

Day, George S. "Diagnosing the Product Portfolio." *Journal of Marketing* 41, no. 2 (April 1977), pp. 29–39.

Hamelman, Paul W., and Edward M. Mazze. "Improving Product Abandonment Decisions." *Journal of Marketing* 36, no. 2, (April 1972), pp. 20–26.

Harrigan, Kathryn Rudie. "Strategies for Declining Industries." *Journal of Business Strategy* 1 (Fall 1980), pp. 20–34.

Harris, John S. "New Product Profile Chart." *Chemical and Engineering News* 39 (April 17, 1961), pp. 110–118.

Henderson, Bruce D. "The Product Portfolio." *Perspectives.* Boston Consulting Group, 1970.

Levitt, Theodore. "Exploit the Product Life Cycle." *Harvard Business Review* 43 (November–December 1965), pp. 81–95.

Robinson, S. J. Q.; R. E. Hichens; and D. P. Wade. "The Directional Policy Matrix —Tool for Strategic Planning." *Long Range Planning* 11, no. 3, pp. 8–15.

Rothe, James T. "The Product Elimination Decision." *MSU Business Topics* 18, no. 4, pp. 45–52.

Wind, Yoram, and Vijay Mahajan. "Designing Product and Business Portfolios." *Harvard Business Review* 59, no. 1, (January–February 1981), pp. 155–165.

Sales:

Churchill, Gilbert A., Jr.; Neil M. Ford; and Orville C. Walker, Jr. *Sales Force Management* Homewood, Ill.: Richard D. Irwin, 1981.

Semlow, Walter J. "How Many Salespeople Do You Need?" *Harvard Business Review,* 37 (May–June 1959.) pp. 126–32.

Steinbrink, John P. "How to Pay Your Salesforce." *Harvard Business Review* 56 (July–August 1978), pp. 116–117.

▨ CHAPTER 8

INTEGRATION OF THE MARKETING PLAN—STEP 5

Step 5 involves the process of integrating the marketing plan into the organization. First, the plan must be integrated with the other major functions of finance, personnel, and operations. Second, the plan has to be integrated within the context of other business plans and programs to make sure that competition is minimized, resources are maximized, and the business is most efficiently managed. This is commonly referred to as portfolio management. As a result of discussions in these two areas, market plans may be accepted, modified, or completely rejected—and the business therefore eliminated.

The process of integration is a dynamic one, based on personalities, politics, available resources, and the tone of the organization. The accomplishment of this step can require the development of a revised marketing strategy, which may be different from the original strategy. A revised marketing strategy often occurs because of resource allocation needs, coordination with other market plans, and the integration of the plan with the organizational mission. This chapter examines the integration of the market plan with other management functions and with the organization's overall portfolio.

Step 5: Integration of the Marketing Plan

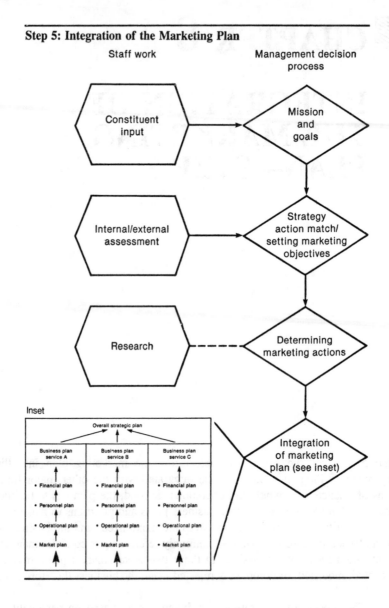

Staff work   Management decision process

Constituent input → Mission and goals

Internal/external assessment → Strategy action match/ setting marketing objectives

Research → Determining marketing actions

Integration of marketing plan (see inset)

Inset

Overall strategic plan

Business plan service A	Business plan service B	Business plan service C
• Financial plan	• Financial plan	• Financial plan
• Personnel plan	• Personnel plan	• Personnel plan
• Operational plan	• Operational plan	• Operational plan
• Market plan	• Market plan	• Market plan

■ Integration of the Proposed Marketing Plans with Other Management Functions

At the outset of this marketing planning process, Exhibit 8–1 indicates that marketing serves as a key first step in the development of a comprehensive business plan. This exhibit was also the starting point in Chapter 3.

As indicated, the marketing plan serves as a basis for the operational plan (i.e., how clinical services will be provided), the personnel plan, and the financial plan (budget, cash management, etc.). Also, marketing plays a

EXHIBIT 8–1
Organization Business Planning Process

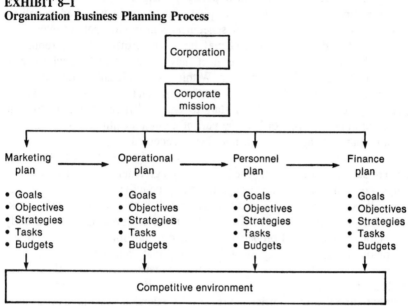

role in helping to formulate overall corporate mission and goals. The scope of marketing includes understanding the environment and connecting the market with the services provided in the hospital or clinic.

While most hospitals and many clinics have people with marketing responsibility, few of them have been able to act as the key agents in developing the business plans. Instead, the more likely scenario is for market data to be analyzed, advertising budgets developed, and sales forecasts made *after* the business has been approved. Many organizations choose to use marketing as a *support* function to decisions initiated in other areas. Marketing provides key input but does not add to the early decisions on service viability. Therefore, an important question which faces marketing in health care is, *to what extent can marketing integrate itself into the organization at a high level, in order to maximize its value?*

Successful health care businesses of the future will have marketing, finance, and operations well integrated in the early stages of service development. Early integration of these functional plans results in a total business plan with a greater likelihood of success. In the following pages, each functional area is briefly examined to better understand its concerns regarding the marketing plan.

Integration with Operations

Operations is concerned with providing clinic or hospital services on a day-to-day basis. As implied in earlier chapters, marketing often means change—

change in service, in location, or in policy. As expected, these changes often affect routine operations. In the hospital, nurses might be asked to call on physician's offices, change work schedules, and modify patient interaction practices. The dietary department may be asked to offer 24-hour room service, while the admissions department may be asked to have physicians' offices linked directly by computer. Within the physician's office, the term "operations" often refers directly to the physician services. A marketing plan may require the physician staff to change office hours, modify the length of appointments, or become part of a clinic health education faculty. Again, change is apparent, but not always accepted.

In order to meet these changes, a variety of operational considerations, such as staffing, equipment, schedules, union agreements, historical relationships, coordination with other departments, productivity analysis, coverage, and call systems must be examined. The result is that many managers ask, why do we need to change? The market plan, if developed without early operations input, would probably be blocked or not implemented in critical operations areas. More important, it is likely that valuable ideas on how to change or establish a competitive advantage in terms of service delivery will be lost. Therefore, instead of going to the family practice department and simply telling them that office hours must be extended, it is more efficient to meet with family practice personnel and show them the consumer research data that indicates a demand for service after normal hours. Viewing the department members as another market segment, the potential impact of this opportunity must be mutually assessed. These individuals can be informally surveyed as to what ideas they might have in designing an after-hours clinic coverage system to capture this business. In this role, marketing serves as a catalyst to integrate organizational direction with the day-to-day provision of service. And, the marketing orientation demonstrates that market segments exist both externally and internally.

Integration with Personnel

Personnel is concerned with providing the proper talent, maintaining a fair system for managing and compensating employees, and developing the appropriate culture within which the organization can develop. As marketing concepts become more widespread, the personnel function will be forced to find solutions to difficult problems. First, personnel will have to find a way to create an entrepreneurial environment within the existing bureaucratic structure of most hospitals. Second, personnel must develop new compensation systems such as bonus plans, commission programs, and incentives. Although common to traditional industries, these alternatives are hardly used in health care. Third, major change in strategy and operations will cause long-standing middle management needs to be reevaluated.

For example, do hospitals need separate departments for ECG, EEG, cardiology, P.T., O.T., and respiratory therapy? Could one manager handle the entire function with well-trained supervisors in each department? Does the hospital need separate department heads for dietary, housekeeping, and admissions or would an executive innkeeper be more capable? A final aspect to consider in the business planning process is top management's needs.

Consider the personnel changes under a more market-responsive system. For example, if a hospital manages the "hotel functions" through an executive innkeeper and the clinical business areas through MBA-trained product (brand) managers, what will come of the assistant administrator function? It is obvious that aggressive marketing plans might cause dramatic changes in all areas relating to personnel.

Most of these changes will take time to be integrated into the organization. Marketing should not develop a market plan in November which calls for the use of commission sales plans for a program manager and expect to get it underway by January. Personnel must be involved in the early sales force planning activity. Alternative compensation systems to reward sales efforts in accordance with organizational goals must be tested.

Personnel will have valuable input for the successful implementation of marketing plans. As with the operations group, marketing should consider personnel a partner in problem solving.

Integration with Finance

Operations is concerned with how to provide quality, efficient service on a day-to-day basis. Personnel maintains human resource systems that match the needs of the organization. Finance is largely concerned with the preservation and growth of capital. To a financial manager, the market plan often represents a degree of risk for which reward should be appropriate.

The higher the perceived risk, the larger should be the return on investment. Finance often evaluates the market plan risks in relation to what can be obtained by investing capital in "safe" areas such as bonds. For example, $1 million invested in a health foods store with no net income for four years is weighed against $1 million in high-grade bonds at 12 percent. The key concern is risk. If a safe return can immediately generate 12 percent return on investment, shouldn't it stand to reason that anything with a higher risk should generate more than 12 percent? The long-term position of the organization, however, may be to extend itself from medicine to health. The short-term loss of the health food store may result in a longer, more profitable position for the organization.

Finance looks at risk in relation to the probability that *targets can be reached, within a reasonable time, and with a large enough return on investment.* Exhibit 8–2 reflects this thinking. From the finance manager's perspective, the risks inherent in most marketing plans are large in relation to a "safe" investment. Can we meet projected sales? Can we control costs? What will the competitors do? What will the economy be like in three years? Do we know this business?

Integrating the finance view is essential to developing effective business (and specifically marketing) plans. Finance is responsible for bud-

EXHIBIT 8–2
Risk/Return Philosophy

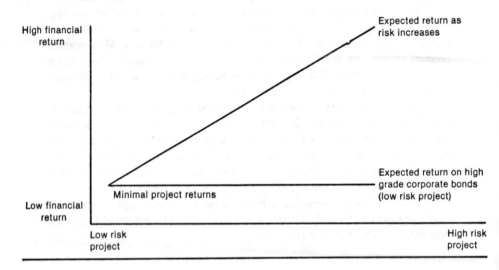

gets, revenue forecasts, and cash flow management. The finance perspective is valuable even beyond these areas. Finance often represents a critical "second opinion," and these experts excel at developing creative strategies to syndicate new ventures. Finance is helpful in weighing risk and evaluating alternative marketing plans.

By nature, finance is often conservative. Its goal is to protect capital from bad risks, and as most financial people know, many ventures are bad risks. Marketing should not try to avoid this critical examination by finance, and it should be particularly encouraged when scarce capital resources exist.

All of the concerns of each functional area are legitimate. Each one needs to be discussed. The key for marketing is to be sensitive to these disciplines, resolve concerns, and understand that marketing is part of a larger business unit upon which success depends.

■ Integration within the Organization's Portfolio

The second aspect of integration relates to the integration of each proposed marketing plan and its related business plan with other proposed marketing plans and business plans. Consider Exhibit 8–3, which was first presented in Chapter 3.

This exhibit shows how each business has a market plan and, taken together, how these plans form the portfolio of activity for the hospital or clinic. The integrative function relates to determining:

EXHIBIT 8–3
The Organization Portfolio

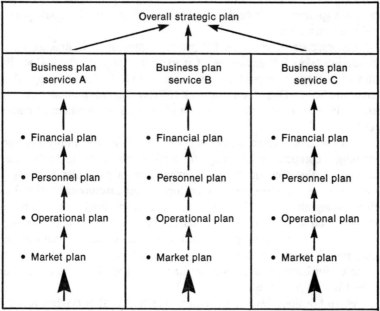

1.   If the proposed plans overlap.
2.   If the proposed plans compete with each other.
3.   If the proposed plans duplicate resources.
4.   If the proposed plans represent the correct balance of activity for the clinic or hospital.

Some examples can help to illustrate what integration between plans means. In 1981, American Express Company purchased the brokerage house of Shearson. With this purchase, American Express was able to offer a full line of financial services. They now provide a financial card through American Express, insurance through Fireman's Fund, and investment advice through Shearson.

Many of these services are directed to upper-income individuals. The American Express Gold Card is an example of this type of offering. Although each business unit has independent responsibility to develop its own marketing and business plans, integration does occur. The company now works on systems to coordinate sales of the three product categories to the same upper-income market segment. The company also explores cross-selling activities. Cross selling refers to the idea of a Shearson broker recommending a Gold Card, and a Fireman's Fund independent agent passing on information about the Shearson brokerage firm. Similar legitimate opportunities exist in health care. For example, an obese patient in the emergency room for a sprained ankle could be given a brochure for a hospital-sponsored weight loss program.

The essence of checking for program integration is making sure the organization takes full advantage of marketplace opportunities. Does home health care support respiratory care? Are OB/GYN doctors supportive of internal medicine? Does the clinic seek to serve the entire family, or is each doctor only concerned with that portion of the family for whom he currently cares?

Prior to this chapter, marketing plans were discussed only as a means of gaining a competitive advantage for a particular program. In the integration process, the concern shifts somewhat from a particular business plan focus to a more complete organization focus. This macroorganizational view includes integration with functional areas, such as finance and personnel, and integration with other business plans. With this more complete organizational focus, the marketing professional and other organizational executives should shift from concern for competitive advantage in a given business plan to concern for balance of the product line, total growth of the organization, and best use of resources.

When hospitals develop plans, are they impartial or do they reflect the strong artificial influence of two or three specialty areas with representatives on the planning committee? Hospitals need to balance their portfolios between sources of business today and sources of business in the future. Often, cash generated from high-profit clinical services will not be invested back into those areas, but into new areas in the hope that they will become the high-profit areas of the future.

Completion of this step and development of the other elements of the business plan will change the original marketing plan. These changes occur as more members participate in refinement of the plan. The final step is to develop a set of game rules for which plans can be approved. This process is developed and explained in Chapter 9.

Checklist for Chapter 8

1. Does this market plan complement the organization and its other services?
2. Do the other management functions complement the market plan?
3. Does the plan provide for a major contribution to the organization?
4. Is the organization spending too much time/effort on this plan for the expected return?
5. As a result of the integration process, do the combined plans offer balance, and are they responsive to the market?

◪ CHAPTER 9

THE APPROVAL AND MONITORING PROCESS—STEP 6

The approval and monitoring process signals the last step in the development of the marketing plan, and the first step in implementation. The marketing job is not over, it is just beginning. Approval of a formal marketing plan begins the attempt to implement the plan. This chapter explores how organizations can select among alternative marketing plans. In order to make this decision, the organization needs a set of guidelines to evaluate alternative plans. This chapter reviews the process of setting guidelines. Moreover, the monitoring process for marketing plans and the need for contingency plans are reviewed. Appendix C provides a complete sample marketing plan in the format outlined in this book.

■ Establishing Guidelines for Selecting among Alternative Plans

Many organizations face the problem of having more ideas and proposed marketing plans than the hospital or clinic can support. Thus, a system to select which marketing plans to implement is needed. In reality, these guidelines represent the "game rules." In actual practice the game rules should be developed in advance of any formal market planning document, and these rules should be available to senior staff as the parameters for business planning. Just as physicians develop criteria for evaluating medical case management before the cases are managed, business plans should be developed after the evaluation criteria have been specified. Prespecification of guidelines has

Step 6: Approval and Monitoring the Plan

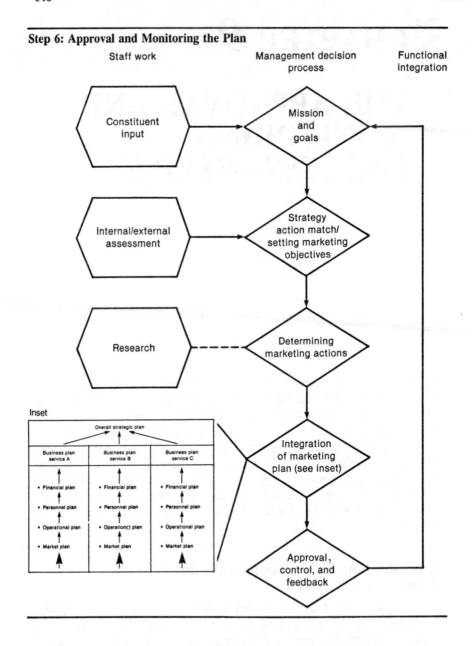

Staff work   Management decision process   Functional integration

Constituent input → Mission and goals

Internal/external assessment → Strategy action match/ setting marketing objectives

Research ⟶ Determining marketing actions

Integration of marketing plan (see inset)

Approval, control, and feedback

Inset

Overall strategic plan

Business plan service A	Business plan service B	Business plan service C
• Financial plan	• Financial plan	• Financial plan
• Personnel plan	• Personnel plan	• Personnel plan
• Operational plan	• Operationcl plan	• Operational plan
• Market plan	• Market plan	• Market plan

several advantages: time is saved by avoiding projects that do not meet predetermined standards, unwise "pet" projects are avoided, and the expectation level required to meet the organization's mission is communicated. In Chapter 7 a chart was presented which guides the selection of *new product offerings*. This same general approach can be used to choose market plans.

As indicated by Exhibit 9–1, a quantitative method can be used to

EXHIBIT 9–1
Evaluation Checklist

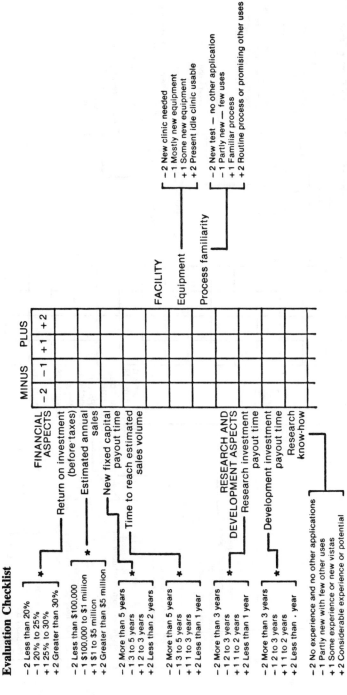

FINANCIAL ASPECTS

Return on investment (before taxes)
- −2 Less than 20%
- −1 20% to 25%
- +1 25% to 30%
- +2 Greater than 30%

Estimated annual sales
- −2 Less than $100,000
- −1 $100,000 to $1 million
- +1 $1 to $5 million
- +2 Greater than $5 million

New fixed capital payout time
Time to reach estimated sales volume
- −2 More than 5 years
- −1 3 to 5 years
- +1 2 to 3 years
- +2 Less than 2 years

- −2 More than 5 years
- −1 3 to 5 years
- +1 1 to 3 years
- +2 Less than 1 year

RESEARCH AND DEVELOPMENT ASPECTS

Research investment payout time
- −2 More than 3 years
- −1 2 to 3 years
- +1 1 to 2 years
- +2 Less than 1 year

Development investment payout time
- −2 More than 3 years
- −1 2 to 3 years
- +1 1 to 2 years
- +2 Less than . year

Research know-how
- −2 No experience and no other applications
- −1 Partly new with few other uses
- +1 Some experience or new vistas
- +2 Considerable experience or potential

FACILITY

- −2 New clinic needed

Equipment
- −1 Mostly new equipment
- +1 Some new equipment
- +2 Present idle clinic usable

Process familiarity
- −2 New test — no other application
- −1 Partly new — few uses
- +1 Familiar process
- +2 Routine process or promising other uses

*The ratings for this aspect will depend on the individual company's type of business, accounting methods, and financial objectives. The values shown above are estimated on the basis of various published information to bracket the averages for large chemical companies.

(continued)

EXHIBIT 9–1 (concluded)

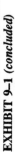
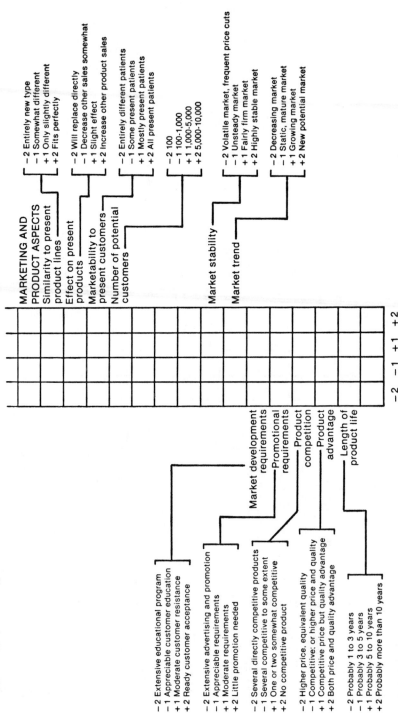

MARKETING AND PRODUCT ASPECTS

Similarity to present product lines
- −2 Entirely new type
- −1 Somewhat different
- +1 Only slightly different
- +2 Fits perfectly

Effect on present products
- −2 Will replace directly
- −1 Decrease other sales somewhat
- +1 Slight effect
- +2 Increase other product sales

Marketability to present customers
- −2 Entirely different patients
- −1 Some present patients
- +1 Mostly present patients
- +2 All present patients

Number of potential customers
- −2 100
- −1 100–1,000
- +1 1,000–5,000
- +2 5,000–10,000

Market stability
- −2 Volatile market, frequent price cuts
- −1 Unsteady market
- +1 Fairly firm market
- +2 Highly stable market

Market trend
- −2 Decreasing market
- −1 Static, mature market
- +1 Growing market
- +2 New potential market

Market development requirements
- −2 Extensive educational program
- −1 Appreciable customer education
- +1 Moderate customer resistance
- +2 Ready customer acceptance

Promotional requirements
- −2 Extensive advertising and promotion
- −1 Appreciable requirements
- +1 Moderate requirements
- +2 Little promotion needed

Product competition
- −2 Several directly competitive products
- −1 Several competitive to some extent
- +1 One or two somewhat competitive
- +2 No competitive product

Product advantage
- −2 Higher price, equivalent quality
- −1 Competitive: or higher price and quality
- +1 Competitive price but quality advantage
- +2 Both price and quality advantage

Length of product life
- −2 Probably 1 to 3 years
- −1 Probably 3 to 5 years
- +1 Probably 5 to 10 years
- +2 Probably more than 10 years

−2 −1 +1 +2

Source: John S. Harris, "New Product Profile Chart" *Chemical and Engineering News*, 39 (April 17, 1961) pp. 114–15. Reprinted with permission, Copyright 1982 American Chemical Society.

evaluate business plans. This approach uses a numerical scoring system. Those plans which score highest are the plans which are approved. Each organization must develop its own criteria and scoring system according to the specific guidelines and needs of the hospital or clinic. Differential weighting of each criterion should be determined by the management and board.

Another approach is to use a less structured evaluative method, concentrating more on the general advantages or disadvantages of one plan over another as illustrated in Exhibit 9–2. In this approach, guidelines are less specific and quantifiable. Instead, the idea is to evaluate general positive and negative attributes of the business plan.

EXHIBIT 9–2
A Qualitative (Less Formal) Approval Process

	Check 1 item per criteria	
Criteria (examples)	+ Positive evaluation	– Negative evaluation
• Return on investment	_____	_____
• Volume of revenue generated	_____	_____
• Competitive advantage	_____	_____
• Location	_____	_____
• Life cycle match	_____	_____
• Available technical know-how	_____	_____
• Financial risk	_____	_____
• Competition ability	_____	_____
Overall evaluation		

For many health care services, decision criteria cannot be provided with quantitative scales such as in Exhibit 9–1. The mix of organizational motivations, which often include the desire to survive as a service as well as more intrinsic motives which relate to community service, goodwill, and the public good, complicate a strict numerical system. Therefore, a more common approach to evaluation is shown in Exhibit 9–2, in which the process is used more as a point of reference for decision making than as a strictly quantitative, evaluative process.

Whatever method is selected, it is important that the method be developed in advance and all plans evaluated against it as suggested in Exhibit 9–3.

This method accommodates differences in return on investment (ROI), investment/risk, and other factors to allow for a rational determination of the mix of plans that makes the most sense. The following is a sample of criteria generally used in the evaluation process.

EXHIBIT 9–3
Selecting Among Alternative Business Plans

Selection criteria*	A Proposed plan Home health + −		B Proposed plan Heart surgery − −		C Proposed plan Vision center + −	
1. Return on equity						
2. Volume of revenue						
3. Competitive advantage						
4. Certificate of need						
5. Capital required						
6. Ease of entry						
7. Research time required						
8. Knowledge of business						

*Examples of possible selection criteria

Return on Equity

One of the most common criteria for evaluating alternative projects involves an analysis of return on equity (ROE). This item refers to the percentage of return realized from the owners' equity. A $1 million dollar investment with a net income of $100,000 translates into a return of 10 percent. Several more precise methods of calculating return are available. Generally, projects which have an average return in excess of 20 percent, over the life of the investment, would score very favorably.

Exhibit 9–4 presents examples of return on equity for several companies. Projects that score an average project life of 10 percent or less would score low. Yet any return on equity must be tied to the organization's cost of capital. As the perceived risk of a project increases, or as the length of time increases before profits are realized, the expected return usually increases. While return on equity represents a good indicator of how well the investment is doing overall, other criteria are also necessary.

Volume of Sales

Small projects or new service offerings can generate large returns on investment. However, many times organizations must look beyond ROE analysis to make sure the project is of sufficient magnitude in terms of absolute gross revenue dollars to add to the organization. An important issue is whether the service generates substantial cash flows which are large enough for management to spend time on them in the first place.

Each organization must determine the exact specification of this criterion. In some hospitals, projects that do not expect to have annual revenues of $1 million within three years would be rejected; whereas in other organi-

---

EXHIBIT 9–4

Net Income as a Percentage of Stockholder Equity

	Percent
American Hospital Supply	19.4
Hospital Corporation of America	13.7
Holiday Inns Inc.	8.1
Dun & Bradstreet	28.2
National Medical Enterprises	16.7
Walt Disney Productions	7.9
Servicemaster	39.4
Citicorp	15.0
Sears, Roebuck & Company	9.8

Source: "The Fortune Directory of the Largest U.S. Nonindustrial (service) Corporations," *Fortune,* June 13, 1983, p. 152.

---

zations, projects which generate gross revenues of $300,000 are considered acceptable.

Return on Sales

Return on sales represents another criterion which is often incorporated into the selection process. Return on sales helps to provide a balanced analysis of the financial value of the market plan, when used in conjunction with the previously mentioned criteria. If an eye glass store has sales of $2 million and profit of $400,000, the return on sales would be 20 percent ($2,000,000 ÷ $400,000 = 20%). The reason it is worthwhile to look at both return on equity and return on sales can best be illustrated by the following example.

A hospital is considering a business plan for a health foods chain and a large retail drug store. The alternative results are as follows:

	Health Food Chain	Drug Store
Sales	$5,0000,000	$5,000,000
Net income	100,000	500,000
Total equity investment	500,000	2,500,000
Return on sales (percent)	2	10
Return on equity (percent)	20	20

The health food store operation has a low gross margin and as a result, generates a relatively small profit on each dollar of sales compared to the drug store. However, because the investment required is lower for the health foods store, the percentage of return in each project is the same. As a result of this analysis, it is apparent that several financial criteria are useful in order to evaluate alternative marketing and business plans.

Existing Competition

An objective evaluation of the number of competitors and the threat they pose is also a useful criterion for plan approval. Clearly, if few competitors exist in a market that is known to be capable of sustaining a clinic office, a business plan suggesting such an action would get a positive score. On the other hand, a business plan which proposes to enter a competitively intense area with few service innovations would get a low rating. Be aware, however, that at times it is a good strategy not to enter the market first. If the service is completely new and untried, it may be useful for someone else to enter first and bear the necessary expense of educating the market. The second entry would be able to learn from the first, avoid some expensive media costs, and catch the market as it moves from the introduction phase to the growth portion of the market life cycle.

Technical Protection

Marketing plans which entail new services or products that have patent protection, regulatory protection, or technical advantages, should be evaluated more positively. Patent protection refers to the exclusive use of a product or service through research and development, and ultimate proprietary rights. This protection is rare in a health clinic setting. Regulatory protection refers to the necessity of obtaining a certificate-of-need before establishing a service. This form of protection has been valuable in the past for health care providers but has diminished with the uncertain future of certificate-of-need regulations. Technical know-how refers to the special capability, equipment, manpower, and other factors that an organization has. It is recognized that others could develop this capability but that it is expensive, risky, and difficult to do. As new technological advances rapidly enter the market, the length of time in which a market plan can be based on this advantage is limited.

Each of these examples represents the type of analysis which should be explored as each individual business plan is considered. Exhibit 9–5 provides an overview of possible criteria to use. In order for the marketing plan and subsequent business plan to develop to the greatest level of precision and potential, the development of defined criteria should be completed before the marketing and business plans are begun.

During this evaluation it is also important to analyze marketing and business plans for logic and consistency. For example, it is difficult to have

---

EXHIBIT 9 – 5
Screening Criteria for Plan Selection

Screening Criteria Can Be Summarized by Asking:
1. Is the return on the investment adequate?
2. Does it enhance political power?
3. Are estimated revenues sufficient and profitable?
4. Does it require capital? To what extent?
5. Does it require research time?
6. Is a certificate-of-need required?
7. Does it have a competitive advantage in the marketplace?
8. Does it have a solid market segment?
9. Is it easy for a competitor to duplicate?
10. Is it a process with which our organization is familiar?
11. Does it enhance stability of the other products offered by the organization?
12. Does it promote product competition?
13. Does it provide for long-range growth?
14. Does it provide for adequate market share?

---

high profits and high growth in the same product in the same year. The growth stage of the life cycle often requires a higher level of expense in the form of capital needs, new staffing, promotion, and general start-up costs. These costs diminish net income in the short term. Also, it is generally not likely that an organization can seek high growth opportunities and at the same time require stability. Aggressive investment in market plans with mature markets is rarely logical. Instead, investment in this type of market condition should be minimized. Generally speaking, this process should review six areas as identified by Jain[1].

1. Internal consistency. (Is the plan consistent with company ideas and direction?)
2. Consistency with the environment.
3. Appropriateness in light of available resources.
4. Satisfactory degree of risk.
5. Appropriate time horizon.
6. Work ability.

These guidelines will help to develop appropriate criteria to aid in implementing those plans which can best serve the agreed upon goals of the organization.

---

[1] Subhash C. Jain, *Marketing Planning & Strategy* (Cincinnati, Ohio: South-Western Publishing, 1981).

■ Monitoring Systems

If the prior steps have been properly followed, a precise, measurable, and targeted market plan will have been developed and approved. The purpose of this book has been to explore methods of developing explicit market plans. The direction of this book is not to examine the day-to-day management of the marketing plan. However, it is appropriate to briefly review the need for monitoring systems designed to help evaluate the effectiveness of the plan and, if necessary, assist in making modifications.

To this point, discussion has concentrated on developing a plan that will have a high likelihood of success. As the organization begins to implement the plan, the use of monitoring systems is necessary. Over the long run, the organization will be monitoring results which are broad in scope. These evaluation systems include return on equity which was discussed earlier in this chapter. Most of the monitoring systems that are specific to a marketing plan are often short term in nature, designed to test, monitor, and, if necessary, adjust marketing plans as needed. The development of these types of day-to-day monitoring systems helps in determining what strategies should be employed in future market plans.

The first monitoring tool, useful to the marketing department and the rest of the organization, is performance in relation to budgeted plan. This system is fundamental to any organization. As Exhibit 9–6 indicates, each month the organization should prepare an income statement which shows: what was planned, (column A); what happened, (column B); the difference between the first and second column, (column C); and actual performance last year (column D).

This exhibit represents a quick and timely snapshot of the performance

---

EXHIBIT 9–6

Home Health, Inc.
Budgeted/Actual Income Statement
May 198__

	(A) Budget	(B) Actual	(C) Variance	(D) Last Year Actual
Sales	$100	$90	$10	$50
Expenses:				
Salaries	$ 50	$51	$ (1)	$40
Travel	4	5	(1)	3
Office supplies	3	2	1	2
Medical supplies	14	20	(6)	10
Rent	3	3	—	2
Utilities	1	1	—	1
Total expenses	75	82	(7)	58
Net income (loss)	$ 25	$ 8	$(17)	$ (8)

EXHIBIT 9–7
Product/Service Sales Analysis (Laboratory)

	Gross Sales	Net Income	Percentage Return on Sales*
Lab test 1	$30	$6	20
Lab test 2	35	6	17
Lab test 3	60	(5)	−8
Lab test 4	50	3	6

*Return on sales $= \dfrac{\text{Net income}}{\text{Sales}}$

---

of a home health business. It shows that profit was achieved for the month and that business has grown since the previous year. It also shows that the level of net income was less than expected due to the problem of lower than anticipated sales and higher than anticipated expenses. This scenario indicates that greater emphasis needs to be placed on the achievement of sales volume. This might occur through the development of a more aggressive sales strategy while holding back operational expenses.

Although this type of expense statement analysis is valuable, other monitoring systems are more specific to the marketing area. First, it is worthwhile to track sales by a specific business or service area.

Exhibit 9–7 shows total sales volume for the month, net income by laboratory test, and the percentage return of profit for each dollar of sales. This format helps to pinpoint those areas which generate strong profits for each dollar of sales and those that are in difficulty.

Lab test 3 has strong sales but has a negative income. This information can be helpful in adjusting prices, eliminating services, or modifying the commission plan to encourage sales in higher margin areas.

Another monitoring tool is required when a sales force is in place. It is helpful to look at the *activity* of each salesperson and the performance or *outcome* of those related sales activities. Exhibit 9–8 provides an analysis of each salesperson, the total sales force, and important productivity measures.

Column A lists the names of each sales person. Column B provides a summary of total sales calls by salesperson and a total for the entire group. Column C provides data on actual sales with column D providing a useful ratio of actual sales to sales calls (Sales ÷ No. of calls = Sales ratio). Column E represents the revenue each salesperson is expected to generate followed by columns F and G which show actual revenue and variance from budget.

This analysis shows that while salesperson K.E. makes many calls, the number of HMO contracts sold is low. On the other hand, salesperson B.M. makes relatively few calls but has a high sales ratio which in turn generates revenues well beyond the budgeted expectation. This indicates that it is

EXHIBIT 9−8
Doctors HMO, Inc. Sales Force Analysis (biweekly)

(A) Salesperson	(B) No. of Calls	(C) Sales	(D) Call to Sales Ratio	(E) Revenue Generated	(F) Revenue Budget	(G) Variance
M.E.	12	1	8%	$ 25	$ 40	$(15)
K.E.	15	0	0	—	40	(40)
B.M.	10	3	30	90	40	50
B.H.	17	2	12	42	40	2
Total	54	6	11%	$157	$160	(3)

necessary to look not only at total sales calls, but also at actual sales and volume of dollars generated in order to get an accurate sales force analysis.

This type of analysis should be done on a monthly basis at a minimum. The data are easy to collect and track, allowing for the quick pinpointing of problem areas and the tracking of individual performance. This information can, in turn, lead to supporting the sales function. Possibly the low producer in Exhibit 9–8 is new and needs to attend educational training. Maybe this person's sales territory is not appropriate or the low producer could learn by spending time with the high producer to observe how higher levels of sales are achieved. In any case, this system allows for fast analysis and concurrent actions designed to meet the objectives of the marketing plan.

In advertising, the determination as to whether or not monitoring systems can be used will be dependent upon the advertising objectives as stated in the action chapter. Some advertising will be directed toward educating potential buyers about a new service or telling consumers how a service can be used. In these cases it may be difficult to tie an ad campaign to immediate sales. When the ads are specifically about a product or service, monitoring becomes more precise and valuable.

Assume that a health foods store located on the first floor of a medical arts building has a campaign in the newspaper with a coupon. A monitoring system could be developed to test which of several different ads (with the coupon) is the biggest draw into the store.

In Exhibit 9-9 three different ads were developed at different costs. Because a coupon was used, it was possible to track the volume of sales that each ad generated. Column B indicates the cost of each ad. Column C indicates the amount of sales attributed to the coupon in each of the three different ads. Column D shows which ad was the most efficient by cost of the ad in relation to volume of sales generated. The small ad cost $.20 for each $1 generated. The medium ad was more efficient in that it cost $.19 to generate $1 in sales. The large ad did not do as well since each $1 of sales cost $.31 in advertising.

When evaluating advertising, numerous monitoring systems can be used. Often it is wise to use several approaches because advertising can be

---

EXHIBIT 9−9
Health Foods Store Advertising Analysis

(A) Ad Description	(B) Cost Per Ad	(C) Coupon Sales per Ad	(D) Ad Costs per $1 of Sales
Small Ad 2 × 10	$1,000	$ 5,000	$.20
Med. Ad 3 × 10	2,000	11,000	.19
Large Ad 4 × 20	4,000	13,000	.31

$$\frac{\text{Cost per ad (col. B)}}{\text{Sales per ad (col. C)}} = \text{Ad cost per \$1.00 of sales (col. D)}$$

---

affected by many variables. For example, the same size ad can generate different responses because of its graphics. Ad impact might also change according to which day it appears in the paper, where in the paper it appears or when it appears on TV and what TV station is used. Advertising agencies are helpful in evaluating which media methods to use, how to monitor ad performance, and when to make changes.

The above monitoring examples represent some of the different ways in which a marketing plan can be evaluated on a continuous basis. The development of specific monitoring systems for a specific service will depend on the strategies used in the market plan.

■ The Need for Contingency Plans

Contingency planning addresses the simple fact that events do not always occur as expected. A few years ago, contingency planning was not at all common. In recent years, however, because of growing uncertainties in an increasingly complex business environment, more organizations have included contingency plans in their planning programs. A contingency plan is based on uncertainty. The premise of a contingency plan is that the outcome of a given situation will *not* be what was expected.

For those organizations that practice contingency planning, the "what if" strategies are usually well thought-out, but the detailed plans of action are not usually as well developed as the primary operating plans. However, the greater the perceived risk of the plan, the more detailed are the contingency plans.

The assumptions portion of the situation analysis is the basis for the development of contingency plans. This section should include the major assumptions/statements regarding the outcome of significant events in which the degree of uncertainty is great, and the risk of being wrong is high.

In the financial area it might be assumed, for example, that inflation for the next three years will average 12 percent per year. If the degree of economic uncertainty is perceived to be high, contingency plans would include the development of financial forecasts. These forecasts might show the impact of the expected rate of inflation *and* a scenario for a higher rate of inflation (e.g., 15 percent) on the plan under consideration.

■ Planning for Next Year

The implementation and use of this year's marketing plan (and entire business plan) for each of the organization's respective service areas, will be a valuable resource for the next year's planning cycle. The monitoring systems and financial statements provide insight as to opportunities in the market, likelihood of reaching profit expectation, competitive turbulence, and the ability to execute marketing plans correctly.

This type of information will help the organization to fine tune its business direction and strategies. Therefore, marketing planning must be both integrated and interactive in nature. The process is integrated in that it works with all elements of the organization. It depends on finance, operations, and personnel. It feeds data to the planning department in order to help set strategic direction. The plan is interactive in that its development depends on feedback, give and take, and constant modification. It is not a process in which finance is involved only temporarily, or where operations contributes only in a prescribed way. Instead, constant input from all areas is required. The cycle of marketing planning and modification is also constant. In this way marketing remains responsive and competitive.

References

Beik, Leland L., and Stephen L. Buzby. "Profitability Analysis by Market Segments." *Journal of Marketing* 37 (July 1973), pp. 48–53.

Dunne, Patrick, and Harry I. Wolk. "Marketing Cost Analysis: A Modularized Contribution Approach." *Journal of Marketing* 41 (July 1977), pp. 83–94.

FitzRoy, Peter T. *Analytical Methods for Marketing Management.* New York: McGraw-Hill, 1976.

Hillier, Frederick S., and David V. Heebink. "Evaluating Risky Capital Investment." *California Management Review* 8 (Winter 1965), pp. 71–80.

Hopkins, David S. "Marketing Performance Evaluation." *The Conference Board Information Bulletin* February 1979.

Hulbert, James M., and Norman E. Tay. "A Strategic Framework for Marketing Control." *Journal of Marketing* 41 (April 1977), pp. 12–20.

Kirplani, V. H., and Stanley S. Shapiro. "Financial Dimensions of Marketing Management." *Journal of Marketing* 37 (July 1973), pp. 40–47.

Mossman, Frank H.; Paul M. Fischer; and W. J. E. Crissy. "New Approaches to Analyzing Marketing Profitability." *Journal of Marketing* 38 (April 1974), pp. 43–48.

Sevin, Charles H. *Marketing Productivity Analysis.* New York: McGraw-Hill, 1965.

▨ CHAPTER 10

CONCLUSION

This book has concentrated on developing a methodology which will allow for the logical development of marketing plans. This methodology begins with the concept of organizational mission and goes through all the essential steps to the final stages of evaluating and controlling the marketing plan. By looking at the entire marketing puzzle in one book, it is possible to take all of the individual pieces, which include concepts such as mission statements, internal analysis, market research, marketing objectives, sales plans, promotion strategies, and finally develop a composite picture of how marketing can operate within a health care organization. With the changes ahead in the marketplace, a good understanding of the total concept of marketing will be essential.

The health care community is going through a kind of marketplace "future shock." Change is coming so fast that it is difficult for organizations to cope. New ideas affecting the marketplace are introduced before other ideas have had time to work. Prospective payment is not well understood, while PPO moves in behind it. What this means is a quickening of marketing dependency in organizations. Clinics and hospitals, which only a few years ago found the concept of marketing distasteful, must now become experts in this area.

The result is that marketing will take on an important role in the health care organization. For many it may well be a flash in the pan. It will often lack logic, not be consumer-driven, not be founded on market research, and not be developed with an eye toward matching strategy ideas and action ideas. The consumer will see ads and brochures—and they will be attractive, but will they be smart marketing?

This book provides a generic, fundamentalist approach to developing marketing plans in health care organizations. It is based on logic, analysis of customer needs, and the important connection between knowing where you are and knowing what to do. This is called the strategy action match. At some point, however, planning stops and action begins. Thus, the marketing plan sets a direction, but it should also be used day in and day out, as conditions change, as a benchmark for future marketing activities. It is not designed to collect dust, or only to be dusted off for next year's plan. Instead, it should be used daily in the pursuit of organizational mission. Therefore, the successful development of marketing plans to meet the changing competitive challenge is based on a balance between solid strategic thinking and a strong dose of logical action tactics.

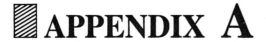# APPENDIX A

CONSOLIDATION OF KEY QUESTIONS USED IN CONDUCTING AN INTERNAL/EXTERNAL ANALYSIS

In Chapter 5, the process of conducting the internal/external analysis was discussed. The internal/external analysis is a key component in developing the marketing plan as it is the foundation from which the strategy action match is determined. It is also key in that it helps to determine which specific action-oriented marketing tactics would be appropriate.

This appendix is a composite of those questions that were first listed in Chapter 5.

■ The Environment and the Market

1. What kinds of external controls affect your organization:
   Local?

   State?

   Federal?

   Self-regulatory?

2. What are the main developments with respect to demography, economy, technology, government, and culture that will affect the organization's situation?

3. Who are the organization's major markets and publics?

4. How large is the service area covered by your market?

5. What are the major segments in each market?

6. What are the present and expected future size profits and characteristics of each market or market segment?

7. What is the expected rate of growth of each segment?

8. How fast and far have markets expanded?

9. Where do your patients come from geographically?

10. What are the benefits which customers in different segments derive from the product: economics, better performance, displaceable cost, etc.?

11. What are the reasons for buying the product in different segments: product features, awareness, price, advertising, promotion, packaging, display, sales assistance, etc.?

12. What is the market standing with established customers in each segment: market share, pattern of repeat business, expansion of customers' product use, etc.?

13. What are the requirements for success in each market?

14. What are the customer attitudes in different segments: brand awareness, brand image (mapping), etc.?

15. What is the overall reputation of the product in each segment?

16. What are the reasons which reinforce the customer's faith in the company and product?

17. What are the reasons which force customers to turn elsewhere for help in using the product?

18. What is the life cycle status of the product?

19. What product research and improvements are planned?

20. Are there deficiencies in servicing or assisting customers in using the product?

■ The Competitive Environment

1. How many competitors are in your industry?
    How do you define your competitors?

    Has the number increased or decreased in the last four years?

2. What is your position in the market (size and strength) relative to competitors?

3. Who are the organization's major competitors?

4. What trends can be foreseen in competition?

5. Are there other companies that might be enticed to serve your customers or markets? This should include conglomerates or diversified companies that might be attracted by the growth, size, or profitability of your markets. Choose the most likely new entries and quiz yourself about what you know about them and their strategies.

6. What about companies on the periphery—those which serve the same customers with different but related products. This might include other pieces of equipment related to yours or equipment that would be included in a broader definition of the market. It is impossible to list all related items, but those of closest proximity should be included.

7. List other products or services that provide the same or similar function. Record the percentage of total market sales for each substitute product.

8. Anticipate product innovations which could replace or reduce the sales of your products. When do you think these products will be commercially feasible? (Note: Information about potentially competitive products can be found by searching the U.S. Patent Office or foreign patent offices.)

9. What are the choices afforded patients?
    In services?

    In payment?

10. Is competition based on a price or nonprice basis?

11. How do competitors (segment/price) advertise?

12. List competitors in other geographic regions or other segments who

do not currently compete in your markets or segments, but may decide to.

13. List customers served by your industry. Note those who may want to move backwards, and consider the reasons why such a move may make sense.

14. List suppliers to your industry; note movement and reasons.

■ The Internal Assessment

1. What has been the historical purpose of your clinic?

2. How has the hospital changed over the past decade?

3. When and how was it organized?

4. What has been the nature of its growth?

5. What is the basic policy of the organization? Is it health care or profit?

6. What has been the financial history of the organization?

7. How has it been capitalized?

8. Have there been any accounts receivable problems?

9. What is the inventory investment?

10. What has been the organization's success with the various services promoted?

11. Is the total volume (gross revenue, utilization) increasing or decreasing?

12. Have there been any fluctuations in revenue? If so, what were they due to?

13. What are the organization's present strengths and weaknesses in:
    Management capabilities?

    Medical staff?

    Technical facilities?

Reputation?

Financial capabilities?

Image?

Medical facilities?

14. What is the labor environment for:
    Medical staff (nurses, physicians, etc.)?

    Support personnel?

    How are weaknesses being compensated for and strengths being used?

■ The Marketing Function and Programs

1. Does the organization have a high-level marketing officer to analyze, plan and implement its marketing work?

2. Are the other persons directly involved in marketing activity able people? Is there a need for more training, incentives, supervision or evaluation?

3. Are the marketing responsibilities optimally structured to serve the needs of different activities, products, markets, and territories?

4. Does the organization's personnel understand and practice the marketing concept?

5. What is the organization's core strategy for achieving its objectives, and is it likely to succeed?

6. Is the organization allocating enough resources (or too many) to accomplish its marketing tasks?

7. Are the marketing resources allocated optimally to the various markets, territories and products of the organization?

8. Are the marketing resources allocated optimally to the major elements of the marketing mix; i.e., product quality, personal contact, promotion, and distribution?

9. Does the organization develop an annual marketing plan? Is the planning procedure effective?

10. Does the organization implement control procedure (monthly, quarterly, etc.) to insure that its annual plan objectives are being achieved?

11. Does the organization carry out periodic studies to determine the contribution and effectiveness of various marketing activities?

12. Does the organization have an adequate marketing information system to service the needs of managers in planning and controlling various markets?

■ Products/Services

1. Complete a list of your organization's products and services, both present and proposed.

2. What are the general outstanding characteristics of each product or service?

3. What superiority or distinctiveness of products or services do you have, as compared to competing organizations?
   What are the weaknesses?

   Should any product be phased out?

   Should any product be added?

4. What is the total cost per service (in use)? Is service over- or underutilized?

5. Which services are most heavily used? Why?
   Are there distinct groups of users?

   What is the profile of patients/physicians who use the services?

6. What are your organization's policies regarding:
   Number and types of services to offer?

   Assessing needs for service addition/deletion?

7. History of major products and services:
   How many did the organization originally have?

   How many have been added or dropped?

   What important changes have taken place in services during the last 10 years?

   Has demand for the services increased or decreased?

What are the most common complaints against the service?

What services could be added to your organization that would make it more attractive to patients, medical staff, nonmedical personnel?

What are the strongest points of your services to patients, medical staff, nonmedical personnel?

8. Have you any other features that individualize your service or give you an advantage over competitors?

■ Pricing Strategy

1. What is the pricing strategy of the organization?
    Cost-plus.

    Return on investment.

    Stabilization.

    Demand.

2. How are prices for services determined?
    How often are prices reviewed?

    What factors contribute to price increase/decrease?

3. What have been the price trends for the past five years?

4. How are your pricing policies viewed by:
    Patients?

    Physicians?

    Third-party payers?

    Competitors?

    Regulators?

5. How are price promotions used?

6. What would be the impact of demand on a higher or lower price?

■ Promotional Strategy

1. Is the sales force large enough to accomplish the organization's objectives?

2. Is the sales force organized along the proper principles of specialization (territory, market, product)?

3. Does the sales force show high morale, ability, and effort? Is it sufficiently trained and motivated?

4. Are the procedures adequate for setting quotas and evaluating performance?

5. What is the purpose of the organization's present promotional activities (including advertising)?

   Protective.

   Educational.

   Search out new markets.

   Develop all markets.

   Establish a new service.

6. Has this purpose undergone any change in recent years?

7. To whom has advertising been largely directed:

   Donors?

   Patients?

      Former.

      Current.

      Prospective.

   Physicians?

      On staff.

      Potential.

8. Is the cost per thousand still favorable?

9. Is it delivering the desired audience?

10. What media have been used?

11. Are the media still effective in reaching the intended audience?

12. Are the objectives being met?

13. What copy appeals have been notable in terms of response?

14. What methods have been used for measuring advertising effectiveness?

■ Public Relations

1. What is the role of public relations?
    Is it a separate function/department?

    What is its scope of responsibilities?

2. Has the public relations effort led to regular coverage?

3. Are the public relations objectives integrated with the overall promotional plan?

4. Are procedures established and used to measure the results from the public relations program?

■ Distribution Strategies

1. What are the distribution trends in the industry?
    What services are being performed on an outpatient basis?

    What services are being performed on an at-home basis?

    Are satellite facilities being used?

2. What factors are considered in location decisions?

3. How important is distribution in establishing a competitive advantage for a particular service?
    Where does the hospital or clinic stand on this component?

▨ APPENDIX **B**

MARKETING RESEARCH METHODS

Occasionally a health care organization realizes that additional data are necessary which are not contained in available records. This realization leads to undertaking marketing research. Exhibit B–1 provides examples of typical market research projects. It is the purpose of the appendix to provide a review of some major alternative data gathering approaches. This is not intended to be a comprehensive guide to conducting marketing research. Important issues of sample size, questionnaire design, and analysis are beyond the scope of this appendix.

This section identifies some of the advantages and disadvantages of each of the more common approaches. Exhibit B–2 contains a summary chart of the major criteria to which each method can be compared.

Personal Interview

The personal interview method is potentially the most expensive of data gathering approaches. The primary reason for its high cost is the need for trained personal interviewers. Skilled interviewers are required to ensure that questions are asked correctly and the same way each time. Since the personal interviewer cannot be monitored while actually conducting the interview, a well-trained person is a prerequisite to collecting data. The personal interview method is difficult to use to collect negative or sensitive information.

EXHIBIT B-1
Examples of Typical Market Research Study Areas and Questions Probed

Example 1: A Study to Select a Site for a New Clinic (not a comprehensive list)
Areas probed should include:

Does respondent have a doctor?
How often is the doctor visited?
Does the entire family use the same doctor?
How satisfied is respondent with:
  Doctor?
  Cost?
  Waiting time?
Does respondent know where proposed new clinic site is located?
Is this new site convenient?
What is the likelihood of visiting a new medical group at this site?
What services should be available in a doctor's office?
How much would respondent expect to pay for a routine visit?

Example 2: A Study to Determine Consumer Satisfaction with a Hospital (not a comprehensive list)

Does respondent have a hospital preference?
Rank this hospital against all other competitors for specific service areas.
What do you like best about this hospital?
What do you like least about this hospital?
If your doctor told you to use this hospital, what would you do?
Have you been a patient or visitor at this hospital?

Example 3: Study of Physicians' Attitudes Toward a Specific Hospital Department (not a complete list)

Rank order this hospital (and competitors) for this department for each of the following:
  Quality.
  Attitude.
  Modern technology.
  Price to patient.
  Convenience.
What do you like best about the department?
What do you like least about the department?
In the next two years, what new services should the department offer?
If the above services were offered, how many more patients would you bring to the hospital?

Because of the lack of anonymity, the individual being interviewed may be more inhibited in expressing opinions to a stranger.

The flexibility of the personal interview method is an advantage. Interviewers can probe respondents for greater depth on their answers. Also, if any forms are to be completed, the interviewer can assist. An additional advantage to personal interviews is the control over respondent selection. That is, the personal interviewer knows who is answering, unlike a

EXHIBIT B−2
Alternative Market Research Approaches

Approach Criteria	Personal Interview	Telephone Survey	Mail Survey	Focus Groups
Economy	Most expensive.	Avoids interviewer travel, relatively expensive, Trained Interviewers needed.	Potentially lowest costs (if response rate sufficient).	Relatively expensive.
Interviewer bias	High likelihood of bias. Trust. Appearance.	Less than personal interviewer. No face-to-face contact. Suspicion of phone call.	Interviewer bias eliminated. Anonymity provided.	Need trained moderator.
Flexibility	Most flexible method. Responses can be probed. Assistance can be provided in completing forms. Observations can be made.	Cannot make observations. Probing possible to a degree.	Least flexible method.	Very flexible.
Sampling and respondent cooperation	Most complete sample possible, with sufficient call back strategy.	Limited to people with telephone. No answers. Refusals are common.	Mailing list problem. Nonresponse a major problem.	Need close selection.

mail survey in which the form might be completed by any household member.

Another strength of this approach is the ability to obtain a complete sample. For example, assume an organization needs opinions of five specific company executives regarding preferred provider organizations. With the personal interview, all five people will eventually be interviewed (although this may require repeated call-back visits and some persistence). The other methodologies do not ensure such sample completion possibilities.

Telephone Interviews

An alternative data gathering approach is the telephone interview. Expense is reduced from the personal interview because of the lack of travel time. And, to some extent there is greater anonymity in this process. Most companies that conduct telephone interviews monitor them to determine whether questions are asked appropriately and data are recorded correctly. An increasing disadvantage to telephone interviewing may be people's attitudes about being interrupted by an unsolicited call. And, consumers are becoming more suspicious about who is calling and the real purpose of the call. Unlike personal interviews, it is easy for the person to terminate a telephone interview at any point just by hanging up the receiver.

Telephone interviews are very advantageous for collecting information quickly. For example, if a clinic ran an advertisement in the Wednesday newspaper for its after-hours clinic, telephone interviews could be conducted Thursday morning to determine how many people noticed the ad. Data can be quickly obtained and appropriate decisions made. Of course, the speed of collecting data is a function of the number of telephone interviewers. However, this method surpasses others on the speed of collecting data.

Mail Surveys

Almost all consumers are familiar with mail surveys of one form or another. Because of the elimination of trained interviewers and the relatively low cost of postage, this can be the most inexpensive method of collecting data. The problem with this approach is the response rate. Rarely do all people who receive a survey return a completed form. A concern is whether those who returned the form are in any way different from those people who did not reply. If surveying the organization's patient population, a comparison of the survey's demographic characteristics to those of the clinic's patient population can be made. This approach can provide some insight as to whether the survey respondents are representative. Or, in a general community survey, respondents' profiles may be compared to the community census breakdowns. When the organization knows who responded and who did not, nonrespondent opinions can be sought through an alternative method. Comparison of the group's responses can then be made. Alternative strategies exist for improving response rates on mail surveys. Follow-up calls with an additional mailing of the survey form often helps. Each successive follow-up wave will improve response rate.

Many organizations have also used incentives to encourage response. Depending on who is being surveyed, and the value of the information, an incentive might consist of a direct monetary payment ($.50, $1, etc.), a premium (a pen, gift certificate) or the chance to win a prize. Response rates also improve as the form becomes easier to complete.

Mail surveys are the most limited approach in terms of flexibility. This factor is both a strength and a weakness. The lack of flexibility means respondents cannot be probed on their responses. It is the rare survey form that would encourage response if, following each question, was a phrase, "Why did you say that?" This lack of flexibility (in the sense that once the question is printed on the form, it cannot be altered or sequentially changed) is an advantage. The organization can be assured that all people will read the same question. When interviewers are used, the possibility exists for them to change the wording or imply meaning through voice intonation.

The anonymity of a mail survey may be one of its strongest advantages. Sensitive information or questions which may lead to negative evaluation may be most easily obtained with this data gathering method.

Focus Groups

An approach gaining increasing popularity in health care research is the focus group. This process consists of a trained interviewer who uses a limited number of probing questions in a group interview. Usually 8 to 12 people participate in the process. Exhibit B–3 contains a sample of four focus group questions presented to consumers to obtain their impressions of hospitals.

The expense of a focus group is really the cost of a trained moderator. This person must have the skills to probe and lead a group without dominating the discussion. Occasionally, people are paid a nominal amount to participate in the one and a half to two-hour sessions.

The focus group allows for maximum probing in a group setting. Depending on the topic under study, the participants may have to be as homogeneous as possible. For example, in conducting a focus group among physicians on ways to improve the hospital, it may be best to have physicians of similar specialties. Mixing physicians from varying specialties might raise issues on certain stations or areas that would not pertain to all participants. Thus, rather than being a group discussion, the focus group could lead to a series of individual interviews in a group setting. Members of a focus group should have similar experiences to allow maximum participation.

The focus group process is often helpful at the beginning of a research study. This process may provide direction for the issues to be explored in a more structured mail or telephone survey. Or, many organizations have

---

EXHIBIT B-3
Hospital Image Study Focusing Questions

1. When people are new to a city, one of the first things they may do is consider where they would go to get hospital care if needed. When you are thinking about hospitals, what things are most important to you?

2. Some time during the past several months, you may have been inside a hospital. In walking around a hospital and speaking with people who work or practice there, what things stand out and tell you that "this place is O.K?"

3. People often get a negative impression of a hospital, the people working there, and the type of place that it is. What things do you look for in a hospital that tell you never to come back?

4. Cost and quality of medical care are important issues. When you are thinking about hospitals that have a reputation for quality, what things are most important in building that reputation?

---

viewed the resulting information as sufficient for certain decisions. It is often valuable to conduct more than one focus group on an issue to ensure that responses received in one session are not unique to the group's composition or dynamics.

INTRODUCTION TO THE SAMPLE MARKET PLAN

■ Situation

Metz Clinic is committed to open several primary care clinics. It has opened Metz Clinic North and Metz Clinic South. The 25 physicians who make up these clinics are heavily oriented toward specialty medicine, including urology, general surgery, neurology, and family practice (eight physicians). Also included are one radiologist and one part-time pathologist. Because of the specialty orientation of the group, the clinic is concerned about maintaining its referral base. The Metz Clinics affiliate almost exclusively with a 450-bed general hospital.

The community of Brighton has 900,000 people, with three hospitals and 525 physicians. Thirty percent of these M.D.'s are in eight major clinics of 10 physicians or more including the Metz Clinic. The suburb in which Metz Clinic South is located has a population of approximately 32,000 (see map).

Two HMOs started three years ago and now subscribe 18 percent of the entire market. The community is stable, with mixed industrial and white-collar activity. Overall hospital admissions have declined slightly in the past three years. All hospitals and the eight major clinics are located within three miles of one another. However, two of the large clinics, including Metz Clinic, have begun major outreach efforts.

Metz Clinic South has been in operation for about one year. This clinic

Map of Brighton and Greentree

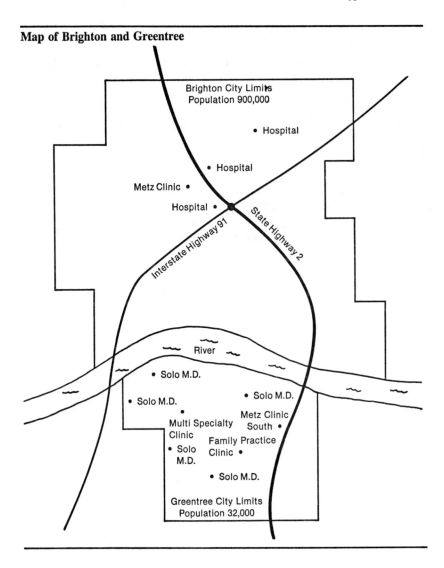

consists of two full-time family practitioners and the equivalent of one additional part-time physician, who maintains half-time obstetrical coverage in Greentree, a suburban community of 32,000 people.

Projected first-year visits of 16,000 to 18,000 did not materialize. Activity only reached 70 percent of this level. Now, as the clinic begins to enter its second year of operation, a marketing plan is completed by the partners and management. The following represents the market plan for Metz Clinic South, located in the suburb of Greentree.

Key areas to focus on while reading the market plan:

1. Notice the extent to which the clinic understands what it is trying to accomplish.
2. Does the clinic understand the environment, the market and the competition?*
3. Does the strategy action match seem logical?
4. Are the marketing objectives specific?
5. Are tactics specific, appropriate, and backed with enough power to meet the marketing objectives?
6. Is the plan logical?
7. Is the plan realistic?
8. Notice the extent to which the plan ties together and the extent to which the logic flows from front to back.

---

*Research provided in the sample plan has been abbreviated from working papers.

SAMPLE MARKET PLAN

Metz Clinic South*
Located in
The Suburb of Greentree

---

*Metz Clinic South—
an outreach clinic of Metz Clinic.
November 198_

TABLE OF CONTENTS

■ I. Introduction and Executive Summary

The purpose of this market plan is to assist Metz Clinic South with growth. The plan will be evaluated at the end of the year. However, modifications of the plan will be made throughout the year as necessary. While this plan concentrates on strategies for the next year, it also establishes a thrust for the next several years.

Metz Clinic South did not meet first-year expectations. Desired performance was not met because of: (1) low visibility; (2) major segments of the population not finding the clinic convenient in terms of hours of service; and (3) a lack of community interest in outreach clinics.

The clinic will modify its operation to attract market segments that want convenience. It will also conduct a promotion program and develop other programs that encourage consumer trial use of the facility. If this differentiation strategy is successful, other clinics within the Metz Clinic organization will adopt these strategies in order to achieve metrowide differentiated recognition through the convenience clinic approach.

■ II. Mission and Goals

A. Mission Statement of Metz Clinic

The mission of Metz Clinic is to provide quality medical and health care services to the greater metropolitan area.

B. Goals of Metz Clinic

1. To be a self-supporting group of physicians involving an appropriate mix of both primary and specialty physicians.
2. To become the predominant medical group in the greater metropolitan area.
3. To provide a broad range of quality services for patients in the area.
4. To maintain a strategy whereby the physician partners achieve incomes which rank in the top one third of all average incomes for physicians in the greater metropolitan area.

C. Additional Goals of Metz Clinic South

To become a five- to seven-physician clinic in Greentree and/or to be the dominant clinic in Greentree.

■ III. Internal/External Analysis Summary

A. The Environment

1. The population of Greentree was 27,000 in 1970 and is 32,000 today.
2. The number of physicians in 1970 was nine and has risen to 16 today.
3. Shopping center growth is rapidly increasing, and housing is lagging.
4. Twenty percent of all clinic patients are government paid (Medicare/Medicaid).
5. Eighty percent of all new health insurance policies written in the greater metropolitan area in the past year involved coverage for second opinions.
6. The population growth appears satisfactory.
7. The available pool of patients also appears satisfactory for the clinic.

B. Market Needs and Segments

1. Forty-eight percent of the community consists of households with people living alone (single, separated, widowed, divorced).
2. Forty percent of all households have a husband and wife both working.
3. Twenty-two percent of all households indicated in market research studies that they would switch hospitals if their doctor selected a hospital they did not like.
4. Each person in this area averages 2.5 visits to a primary doctor per year.
5. Sixty-five percent of all people are under age 55.
6. Fifty percent of the market drives seven miles to the metropolitan area to visit doctors at the "parent clinics."

Market Segment Introduction	Percent of Greentree Population	Percent of Metz Clinic South Practice
1. Women	54%	64
2. Two-income households	40	12
3. Over 50	35	19
4. People who perceive need for comprehensive care	41	45
5. People who seek convenience	65	30
6. HMO patients	12	0

C. Competition

1. One three-person chiropractic clinic exists in the community, and 10 percent of the market "regularly visits."
2. There is one seven-person multispecialty clinic that the market views as the major clinic in this suburb.
3. Five solo practitioners practice in the community.
4. One four-person family practice clinic is in the community and has existed there for over 20 years.
5. Of the 32,000 people in the community, 12 percent are in an HMO obtaining service in the metropolitan area.
6. The major disadvantage that the market perceives regarding the seven-person multi-specialty leader is that they are too busy and difficult to get in to see.
7. The major advantage of the seven-person multi-specialty group is that they are relatively large, well-known and have a good clinical base at this site and at their downtown clinic.
8. The major disadvantage uncovered through market research is that Metz Clinic *South* lacks recognition.

D. Internal Assessment

1. The net income of the partners dipped 4 percent last year, due to the opening of the new outreach clinics.
2. Receivables have increased 30 percent within the past two years.
3. The partners are satisfied with the composition and responsiveness of the professional staff, patient satisfaction, and the service area within which they are practicing.
4. The staff is not satisfied with utilization of the outreach clinic or with its financial condition, due to less than anticipated first-year use.
5. The staff believes that the location and convenient traffic pattern of the outreach clinic are better than what the competitors offer.
6. In the area of visibility within the community, financial condition, and coverage, the clinic is probably not performing as well as the competition.
7. With regard to quality of service, the clinic is performing equally to the competition.

E. Sample Market Research Documentation

TABLE 1
Sample Characteristics

Age		Number of People in Household	
35 and under	40.5%	1	26.5%
36−55	23.5	2	30.0
Over 55	35.5	3 or more	43.5

Religious Affiliation		Length of Time in Neighborhood	
Catholic	47.0%	Less than 5 years	35.0%
Protestant	32.5	6 to 10 years	18.0
Jewish	2.5	More than 10 years	47.0
Other	3.0		
No formal affiliation	13.0		
Refused	2.0		

Age by Area	*Greentree Areas*			
	1	*2*	*3*	*4*
35 and under	44.3%	27.2%	35.5%	34.7%
36−55	21.5	24.3	12.9	30.4
Over 55	33.9	48.5	51.6	34.9

F. Additional Research Questions and Results:

Q: Where do you obtain your medical care and how satisfied are you with your care?

Clinic Used	Percent of Greentree Population Who Use	Percent of Users Very Satisfied
Metz Clinic South	9	87
Metz Clinic	1	(²)
Solo A	2	95
Solo B	4	82
Solo C	1	‡
Solo D	1	‡
Sole E	—	—
Group A	14	81
Other metro clinics*	38	72
No doctor⁺	30	—
	100%	

*Includes HMOs.
⁺Many use chiropractors.
‡Not a large enough sample.

Q: If a doctor's office in Greentree would offer clinic services after business hours, how likely is it that you would visit that office?

	Sample Total	Single Parent	Dual Working Households	Over 65
Very likely	15%	25%	22%	10%
Somewhat likely	25	30	34	15
Somewhat unlikely	30	20	21	50
Not likely at all	30	25	23	25
	100%	100%	100%	100%

Q: What is your insurance coverage?

TABLE 2
Health Insurance Status

Plan	Percentage
Company plan	23.8
Blue Cross	21.8
Health, Inc.	17.1
Medicare	15.5
Shield	3.6
BDB	1.0
M.D. Center	1.0
Other	21.8
Don't know	3.6
Refused	4.1

■ IV. Strategy Action Match and Strategy Selection

It would appear that the marketplace within which the Metz Clinic South is located is growing slightly, but apparently entering a mature stage on the life cycle chart. In addition, the clinic is in an introduction and growth stage, due to the fact that it is only one-year-old and operating at far less than capacity. Therefore, the key strategy for the clinic is to continue to grow, but also to differentiate its service relative to the competition (i.e., offer special or unique services to key segments).

Strategy Overview

A differentiation strategy calls for identifying key segments that need to be served, and establishing a competitive advantage or a series of competitive advantages that make this clinic more attractive to customers than other alternatives.

■ V. Marketing Objectives

Objective 1: Increase clinic visit volume from 12,500 this year to 22,700 by the end of the next fiscal year.

Objective 2: Concentrate on attracting two major segments within the Greentree community. These segments include the segment that is looking for convenience and the segment that contains households where all adults are working. (This would include single, separated, widowed, divorced, and two-income households.)

Objective 3: Increase level of awareness to the extent that 70 percent of each of the target market segments is aware of the clinic and its capability by the end of the second quarter of the next fiscal year.

Objective 4: Reach break-even point by the end of the third quarter of the next fiscal year.

Objective 5: Establish a clear differential advantage for consumers in the community (convenience in location, scheduling, hours of operation, and payment options).

■ VI. Marketing Strategies

A. Service Strategies

1. Expand hours from 10 A.M. to 9 P.M., Monday through Saturday, to attract and accommodate the working market.

2. Provide for unscheduled visits after 5 P.M. (For example, set up a walk-in approach.)
3. Provide a two-hour, midday, unscheduled time for patients with urgent care problems.
4. Increase visibility of staff by providing one doctor- or nurse-developed seminar per month to community or public service groups within the suburb of Greentree.

Responsibility. Assignment of this strategy will be given to Dr. Jones, a medical partner in this clinic.

Cost. Cost for this program will cover a half-time RN and a half-time receptionist ($18,000). Physician coverage will be supported by rotating partners from the downtown clinic.

Expected outcome. It is expected that an additional 3000 visits will be achieved during the first two quarters of the next fiscal year, with the help of these changes.

Completion date. All items are to be completed by the end of the first quarter.

B. Promotion Strategies

1. Establish a copy platform differential advantage which easily explains the new clinic hours and scheduling (i.e., always ready, quick care, urgent care).
2. Construct a back-lit sign, 16 feet high, which uses copy platform concept. Include a lighted "clinic is open" sign.
3. Do a quarterly direct mail to target households regarding availability of service at this site *and* through the main clinic.
4. Place a monthly clinic information stuffer in each patient bill.
5. Coordinate a logo and name identification program to help explain availability.

Responsibility. Advertising agency with clinic manager.

Cost.
a. Agency consulting fee, $6,000.
b. Sign, $14,000.
c. Direct mail program, $8,000.
d. Monthly billing stuffer, $5,000.

Expected outcome.

a. Achieve target patient volume.

b. Achieve 70 percent community awareness of clinic by major market segment.

Completion dates. Steps 1 and 5, January; step 2, March; steps 3 and 4, ongoing.

C. Pricing Strategies

1. Begin to accept credit cards in order to enhance convenience and control accounts receivable.
2. Explore contract with HMO to cover HMO after-hours care.
3. Offer family discount of 10 percent if more than three family members visit per month or if one familly member visits three times per month, to encourage family use.

Responsibility. Clinic manager.

Cost. To be determined.

Expected outcome. New volume, reduction of accounts receivable and more improved income.

Completion dates. Step 1, first quarter; step 2, third quarter; step 3, first quarter.

D. Distribution Strategy

The main strategy is new hours of operation. If this differential advantage of convenience causes activity to grow, the major elements of this plan will be implemented at the other clinics within the system, under a common brand-name strategy. This, of course, will have the effect of a second differential advantage—numerous locations operating under one brand name to provide neighborhood service.

Another advantage of this strategy is that it allows for efficient and more aggressive advertising, plus the option of providing HMO services in an attractive fashion. This is because of geographic spread within the community with retention of a common brand name.

■ VII. Organization and Staffing

A. Organization

Several members of the clinic staff will participate in implementation of the plan. The clinic administrator will be responsible for the overall plan.

B. Staffing

	Current Year	Next Year
Physician	2 FTE	2.3 FTE*
Physicia/OB	.5 FTE	.5 FTE
Office	2 FTE	2.5 FTE*
Technical	3 FTE	3.5 FTE*
	7.5 FTE	8.8 FTE

*Staffing hours will be modified to cover new hours.

■ VIII. Budget: Sample Forms

METZ CLINIC SOUTH
Monthly Operating Statement

	Budgeted	Actual
Revenue:		
Patient visits		
Ancillary	_____	_____
Total revenue	_____	_____
Expenses:		
M.D. salaries		
M.D. benefits		
Staff salaries		
Staff benefits	_____	_____
Sub-total	_____	_____
Office supplies		
Medical supplies		
Discounts		
Utilities......................	_____	_____
Sub-total	_____	_____
Total expenses........	_____	_____
Net revenue..................		
Less: Depreciation		
Net income, before taxes ...	_____	_____

198___ Operating Assumptions

	Actual	Budgeted					Budget Total 198___	Budget Total 198___	Budget Total 198___
		1st Qtr.	2nd Qtr.	3rd Qtr.	4th Qtr.	Total			
# Patient visits									
$ Avg. charge									
Avg. visits/day									
# M.D. staff									
# Staff									
% Medical									
% BX									
Expense cost per test									

METZ CLINIC SOUTH
Projected Operating Statement

	Actual 198__	Budgeted 1st Qtr.	Budgeted 2d Qtr.	Budgeted 3d Qtr.	Budgeted 4th Qtr.	Budget Total 198__	Budget Total 198__	Budget Total 198__
Revenue								
Expenses: Salaries								
Supplies								
Net income								

■ IX. Contingency Plan

If the program fails to show substantial growth by the third quarter, two options will be explored:

1. Selling the practice to another group.
2. Closing the practice and selling the facility.

▨ INDEX